HYDROCEPHALUS
SHUNT
INFECTIONS

HYDROCEPHALUS SHUNT INFECTIONS

ROGER BAYSTON

SENIOR LECTURER IN BACTERIOLOGY
Department of Paediatric Surgery
Institute of Child Health
University of London

HONORARY BACTERIOLOGIST
National Hospital for Nervous Diseases
Queen Square, London

LONDON
CHAPMAN AND HALL

First published in 1989 by
Chapman and Hall
11 New Fetter Lane, London EC4P 4EE

© 1989 R. Bayston

Typeset in 10/12½ Aster by
Scarborough Typesetting Services
Printed in Great Britain at
The University Press, Cambridge

ISBN 0 412 31240 9 hardback
ISBN 0 412 31250 6 paperback

British Library Cataloguing in Publication Data

Bayston, Roger
    Hydrocephalus shunt infections.
    1. Man. Hydrocephalus. Surgery. Shunting.
    Sequelae. Infection.
    I. Title
    617'.514

    ISBN 0–412–31240–9
    ISBN 0–412–31250–6 Pbk

CONTENTS

Acknowledgements   vii

Preface   viii

Foreword   ix

1 Introduction   **1**
  1.1 History of cerebrospinal fluid shunting   1
  1.2 Cerebrospinal fluid shunting devices   3
  1.3 Insertion of cerebrospinal fluid shunts   4
  1.4 Revision of cerebrospinal fluid shunts   10
  1.5 Emergence of septic complications   11

2 Aetiology of shunt colonization   **12**
  2.1 Incidence of shunt colonization   12
  2.2 The nature and classification of shunt
      colonization   13
  2.3 Sources of organisms causing shunt colonization   27
  2.4 Procedures used for characterizing and typing
      bacteria involved in shunt infections   31
  2.5 Shunt infections due to organisms other than
      staphylococci   35
  2.6 Ventriculitis   50
  2.7 Cystic blockage in ventriculoperitoneal shunts   51
  2.8 Summary   56

3 Diagnosis of shunt infection   **58**
  3.1 Clinical features of shunt colonization   58
  3.2 Shunt nephritis   62
  3.3 Other manifestations of immune complex disease   66
  3.4 Laboratory procedures   68
  3.5 Summary   88

4 Surveillance of patients at risk   **90**
4.1 Surveillance scheme   91
4.2 Summary   94
4.3 Recommendations for current practice   95

5 Treatment of shunt infections   **97**
5.1 Alternative treatments   97
5.2 Shunt removal   102
5.3 Shunt removal and immediate reshunting   105
5.4 Antimicrobials   107
5.5 Cell-wall-active antimicrobials   109
5.6 Intraventricular antibiotics   110
5.7 Oral and systemic antimicrobials   110
5.8 Aminoglycosides   114
5.9 Vancomycin   117
5.10 Recommendations for current practice   123

6 Prevention of shunt infections   **126**
6.1 Introduction   126
6.2 Preparation of the patient's skin for operation   126
6.3 Preoperative scalp shaving   128
6.4 The use of drapes   129
6.5 The use of antiseptic barriers at wound edges   130
6.6 Prophylactic antibiotics   131
6.7 Studies using systemic antibiotics   132
6.8 Studies using intraventricular antibiotics   136
6.9 Prophylaxis for dental surgery   138
6.10 Antibacterial catheters   139
6.11 Recommendations for current practice   140

References   141

Index   157

ACKNOWLEDGEMENTS

I owe a debt of gratitude to most of those with whom I have worked, but I must thank especially Professor John Emery, Professor Robert Zachary, Professor David Milner and Professor John Lorber, all of whom taught me a great deal while I worked at Sheffield Children's Hospital.

Much of my own research in this field would not have been possible without the support, financial and otherwise, of the Association for Spina Bifida and Hydrocephalus and its branches.

I would also like to thank my successive secretaries, Samia Shonuga, Marion Ellis and Roz Sullivan for typing and retyping the manuscript.

I am fortunate that my wife, as well as taking more than a fair share of family work and fitting this, not without difficulty, into her own busy professional life, also made many helpful suggestions.

PREFACE

Cerebrospinal fluid shunts, and particularly the problems arising from their use still present an enigma to many groups of health-care personnel. This obviously detracts from the quality of patient care, as well as leading to well-intentioned but misguided research. Having said this, the understanding of shunting and its problems has increased in recent years. However, I feel that there is a need to assess what we now know, as well as what we think we know, in order to take advantage of this understanding and point the way ahead.

I also feel that there are gaps in understanding between the main disciplines, the surgical, the medical and the laboratory, which ought to be bridged if at all possible in order to enhance the quality of service given to our patients who require shunting procedures. In this book I have attempted to address these problems, taking a critical or analytical approach to dogma where necessary, and including information which to some disciplines may appear basic, in order to find common ground with other professional groups. I hope my colleagues will not be discouraged by this approach, leading as it does to some degree of restatement, but will accept that a greater understanding of the roles of one's colleagues in this difficult area can only be beneficial.

R. BAYSTON

FOREWORD

Since its introduction nearly thirty years ago, shunting for hydrocephalus has amply proved its worth as a method of control of excessive collection of cerebrospinal fluid. However, a high proportion of patients remain shunt-dependent for many years and probably permanently, so that it is essential that the chosen method of control is safe and can be maintained indefinitely. Shunt infection has proved to be one of the most troublesome complications, leading to heavy morbidity and significantly increased overall mortality. Though much has been written on the subject, diagnosis and treatment have remained haphazard and ineffective in many centres.

This book is the first attempt to bring the whole subject together in a comprehensive way. Dr Bayston is ideally fitted to make the attempt. He has had a unique experience of the bacteriology of shunt infections, first in Sheffield, one of the centres pioneering the modern treatment of hydrocephalus, and latterly in the Institute of Child Health in London where he has established a laboratory capable of offering a nationwide reference service. He has shown that, by taking proper precautions and undertaking adequate follow-up, it is possible to reduce the incidence of colonization to modest proportions, and almost eliminate its serious and potentially fatal late complications.

Besides a profound knowledge of the complex microbiology involved, the author brings a wide understanding of the clinical problems which greatly complicate overall management of colonization whenever it arises. This book will therefore be not only essential reading for microbiologists, but also a regular source of reference for all clinicians involved in the management of hydrocephalic patients as well as paramedical and lay persons concerned with their daily care.

D. M. FORREST

ix

The 'contents' of this book do not necessarily reflect the opinion of Eli Lilly.

1

INTRODUCTION

1.1 HISTORY OF CEREBROSPINAL FLUID SHUNTING

Hydrocephalus has been defined in a variety of ways, but it may conveniently be thought of as a pathological increase in the volume of the cerebral ventricular system due to accumulation of cerebrospinal fluid. This usually results from obstruction in the pathways by which the fluid passes from one ventricle to another or leaves the ventricular system, but there are numerous causes of this obstruction, such as intracranial haemorrhage, purulent meningitis, tumours and congenital anomalies such as the Arnold–Chiari malformation associated with spina bifida. The increase in cerebrospinal fluid volume leads to a rise in intracranial pressure with compromise of cerebral blood flow and stretching of neural tissue, which causes neurological damage resulting in a range of effects from the completely subclinical to blindness, spasticity, dementia and death from respiratory failure.

While drugs such as acetazolamide (Birzis, Carter and Maren, 1958; Tschirgi Frost and Taylor, 1954; Huttenlocher, 1965) and isosorbide (Hayden, Foltz and Shurtleff, 1968; Lorber, 1973; Wise, Mathis and Wright, 1966) and compressive head bandaging (Epstein, Hockwald and Ransohoff, 1973; Porter, 1975) have been used in attempts to control hydrocephalus, the usual approach is to relieve the raised intracranial pressure by drainage of cerebrospinal fluid into another body cavity. Various body cavities have been utilized in the past. Harsh (1954) described the shunting of cerebrospinal fluid from either the fourth ventricle or the spinal subarachnoid space, into the fallopian tubes.

The ureter was utilized by Drachter (1925), Heile (1925) and Matson (1949), and the mastoid antrum by Nosik (1950). A new problem encountered with ureteral shunting which was not found when shunting the cerebrospinal fluid to other sites was the loss of electrolytes, as the fluid was excreted with the urine. Shunting into the peritoneal cavity was first attempted by Ferguson (1898) using implanted silver wire to form a conduit. This relied on the formation of a fibrin sheath around the wire. Other attempts were made to establish lumbar–peritoneal drainage before the use of rubber tubing by Kausch (1905) to form a ventriculoperitoneal shunt. Silver wire was again used by Hartwell (1913) to form a conduit from spinal theca to peritoneum, and this appeared to be successful, the conduit remaining patent until the patient's death two years later from a cerebral tumour. Various other means of establishing drainage into the peritoneal cavity were tried, but were abandoned because of complications consisting mainly of blockage at the distal end by adhesions. Attempts were made to drain fluid from the cerebral ventricles to the large venous sinuses (Payr, 1908; Haynes, 1913) but these were unsuccessful because of thrombosis in the sinuses and retrograde flow of blood into the ventricular system.

The failure of both peritoneal and venous shunts due to blockage was probably a consequence of the use of materials such as natural rubber or polyethylene which are not sufficiently biocompatible. The use of medical-grade silicone rubber for shunting significantly decreased the incidence of failure of ventriculoperitoneal shunts due to adhesions.

The shunting of cerebrospinal fluid into the venous system was also made possible by the relative freedom from thrombosis and by the use of a flow-control valve in a silicone rubber system (Nulsen and Spitz, 1951; Pudenz *et al.*, 1957; Nulsen and Becker, 1965; Becker and Nulsen, 1967).

Nowadays, all cerebrospinal fluid shunts are made from medical-grade silicone rubber, sometimes with the addition of stainless-steel components. The drainage routes commonly used are from cerebral ventricle to right cardiac atrium (ventriculo–atrial) by way of the neck veins, and from cerebral ventricle to peritoneal cavity (ventriculoperitoneal) using a subcutaneous tunnel over the rib cage. Ventriculopleural and lumbar–peritoneal shunting are also sometimes carried out. When a shunt fails it may be impossible to use the same site for a replacement, and in those patients whose shunts have repeatedly failed, fluid can be shunted from the cerebral ventricles directly into the right cardiac atrium rather than by way of the major vessels (Overton *et al.*, 1967; Blazé, Forrest and Tsingoglou, 1971; Fischer *et al.*, 1972; Tabara, Azmy and Forrest, 1980).

1.2   CEREBROSPINAL FLUID SHUNTING DEVICES

There is now an assortment of shunts available commercially, but they differ little in principle. Apart from the valvular components, there is an array of pumping chambers, antisiphon devices, 'on/off' switch devices (Figure 1.5) and sampling chambers, and two versions of magnetically reprogrammable valves whose flow rates can be changed non-invasively at will.

The most important accessory from the point of view of infection is the Rickham reservoir (Figure 1.1), which, if fitted, allows the removal of ventricular fluid for evaluation and the injection of drugs without repeatedly piercing the brain. Some workers prefer to insert a reservoir separately from the shunt system.

The valvular components are designed to control the rate and direction of flow. They may be slit valves, ball valves or others such as orifice valves. The valves may be situated at the distal end of the

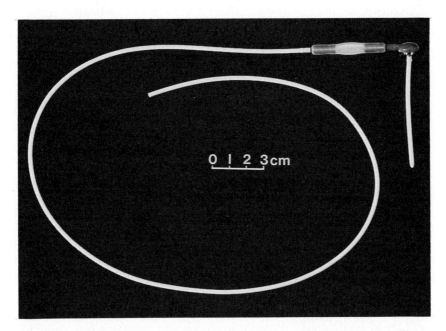

Figure 1.1 Holter valve and Rickham reservoir. There are two unidirectional slit valves each exerting flow control. They are made of silicone rubber and are condom-shaped, being seated in the metal housing. The Rickham reservoir is optional and the distal catheter is fitted separately.

shunt, as in the Raimondi and Unishunt (Figures 1.3 and 1.4) or they may lie in the central portion as in the Holter, Hakim, Multipurpose and Accuflo shunts (Figures 1.1, 1.2, 1.5 and 1.6) and the programmable Medos and Sophy valves. The Holter and Accuflow shunts are the ones most commonly used in the UK, but others promise to increase in popularity.

1.3 INSERTION OF CEREBROSPINAL FLUID SHUNTS

In order to appreciate some of the problems relating to cerebrospinal fluid shunt infections, it is necessary to describe briefly the techniques for implanting a ventriculo–atrial and a ventriculoperitoneal shunt. The Holter shunt is used as an example.

The areas of the planned incisions are prepared and drapes are applied as recommended (see Chapter 6). A curved incision is made in the scalp behind the ear, and the flap reflected with haemostasis as required. A burr hole is then made in the skull and the bone edges trimmed. A 'bed' is made in the skull to receive the valve chamber. A small incision is made in the dura and the ventricular catheter is inserted and positioned, sometimes under radiological control, so that free flow of fluid is obtained. The catheter is then clamped and a retaining suture is inserted, and the site is covered with a gauze pad which may be soaked in an antiseptic such as aqueous povidone-iodine or chlorhexidine. The technique then differs according to whether a ventriculo–atrial or ventriculoperitoneal shunt is to be inserted. In the case of a ventriculo–atrial shunt, an incision is made in the neck and a suitable vein, usually the internal or external jugular, is located. The venous catheter is inserted into the vein and passed into the cardiac atrium. Positioning is checked, either radiographically, by pressure measurements, or by ECG observation, and blood is withdrawn with a syringe to ensure patency (except where distal slit valves are used). The catheter is then clamped and pushed subcutaneously up into the scalp incision. The valve assembly, after testing for correct function, is secured in the prepared 'bed' in the scalp and connected to the ventricular and atrial catheters, using ligatures to secure the connections. A detailed account of a method of insertion of a Holter ventriculo-atrial shunt is given in Tsingoglou and Forrest (1971a).

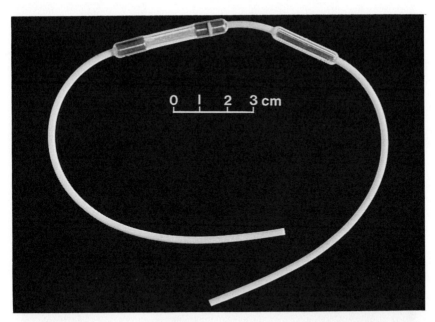

Figure 1.2 Hakim valve. This is superficially similar to the Holter valve but the two valves consist of a sapphire ball seated in a steel cone. The ball opens against a spring which holds it in place against the cone and exerts the force which governs flow rate. The ventricular and distal catheter, reservoir and valve chamber are integral and separate items need not be added, though an extension to the distal catheter is usually necessary.

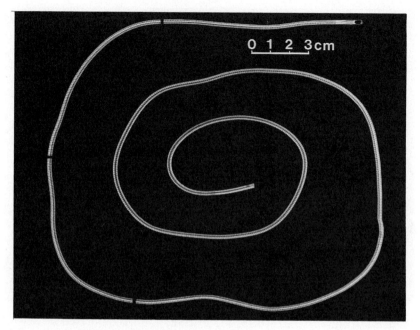

Figure 1.3 Raimondi catheter. This consists of a silicone rubber catheter with a steel spiral embedded in the luminal surface to prevent kinking. A ventricular catheter and preferably a Rickham reservoir must be added. Flow control is exerted by the slit valves at the distal tip.

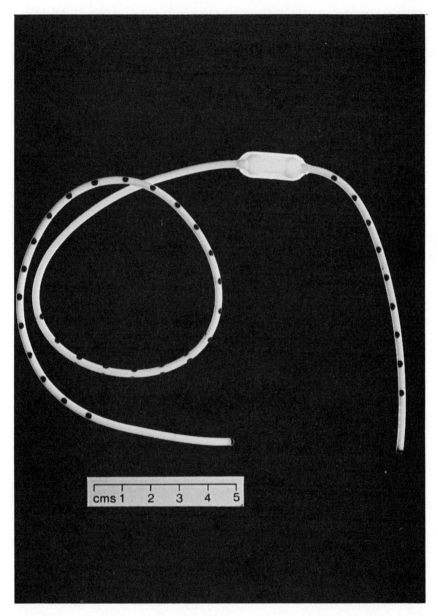

Figure 1.4 Unishunt. This is a single unit with no connections. The valve slits are at the tip of the distal catheter and there is an integral reservoir.

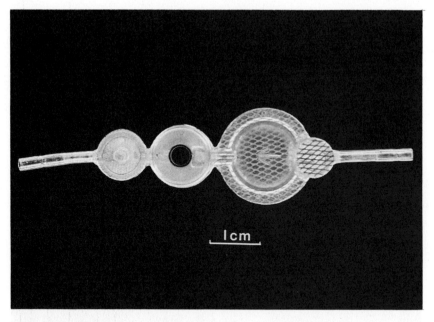

Figure 1.5 Multipurpose valve. This rather complex system involves a reed valve for flow control and an anti-syphon device which is said to prevent slit ventricle formation. There is also a sampling chamber and a switch to turn flow on or off. This is operated by digital pressure through the scalp. Proximal and distal catheters must be connected during insertion.

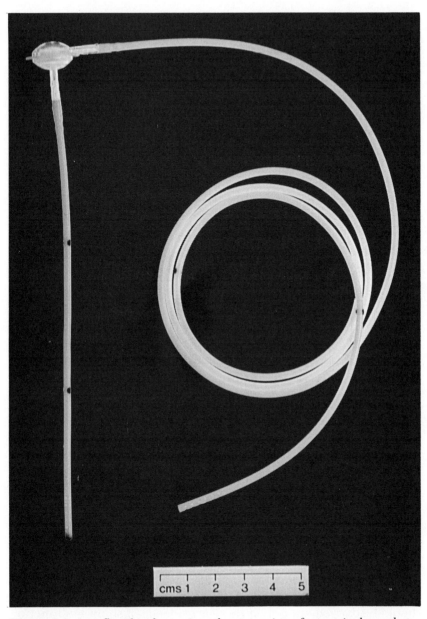

Figure 1.6 Accuflo. This three-piece shunt consists of a ventricular catheter, a diaphragm valve in a domed reservoir, and an open, un-valved distal catheter.

In the case of a ventriculoperitoneal shunt, an incision is made in the neck and another in the abdomen, and the distal catheter is pushed subcutaneously using an introducer from the scalp incision via the neck to the abdominal incision, where it is introduced into the peritoneal cavity. Alternatively, the distal catheter may be pushed from the abdominal incision up to the neck. The components of the system are then connected as in the case of a ventriculo–atrial shunt, and the incisions are closed. It must be emphasized that this is a description of a stylized technique, and many variations are practised. In addition, some surgeons prefer to work in pairs, one at the head and one at the abdomen. For further details of techniques reference should be made to textbooks of operative neurological surgery, and manufacturers' instructions.

The use of a single unit shunt which does not require connections to be made has been described by Raimondi, Robinson and Kuwamara (1977).

1.4 REVISION OF CEREBROSPINAL FLUID SHUNTS

Shunts may be revised by removing one or all components and replacing with new ones, or in some cases by removing the components and replacing them after testing has shown their function and patency to be acceptable, though this latter method is not to be recommended as it greatly increases the risk of shunt infection. Often malfunctioning shunts are revised by re-routing the distal catheter from the venous system into the peritoneal cavity, or less commonly the reverse. When ventriculo–atrial shunts are used in small infants, the distal tip may be pulled out of the atrium and into the superior vena cava as the child's body length increases. The rate of blood flow past the tip decreases and allows partial or total blockage by walling off the catheter. This process also sometimes leads to disconnection or fracture of the distal catheter. For these reasons revision of the distal catheter is frequently required when the child reaches the age of 12 to 18 months. Surgical opinion varies as to whether lengthening should be carried out only if there is evidence of shunt malfunction, or whether it should be carried out prophylactically on all such children when the tip of the distal catheter is seen by X-ray to have risen out of the right atrium (Tsingoglou and Forrest, 1968). In view of the risks of revision and the knowledge that many children with 'non-functioning' shunts remain asymptomatic for long periods, elective revision in the absence of symptoms is not recommended.

1.5 EMERGENCE OF SEPTIC COMPLICATIONS

Holter shunts were first used in the UK in 1958, for ventriculo–atrial shunting, and gradually gained popularity. However, reports began to appear of persistent bacteraemia in patients who had had shunts inserted (Anderson, 1959; Carrington, 1959; Schimke *et al.*, 1961; Cohen and Callaghan, 1961; Callaghan, Cohen and Stewart, 1961; Bruce *et al.*, 1963; Luthardt, 1970; Shurtleff, Foltz and Christie, 1971; Tsingoglou and Forrest, 1971b). Other workers later recorded infections in ventriculoperitoneal shunts (Little *et al*, 1972; Bayston and Spitz, 1977). The organisms involved in both types of shunt were usually staphylococci, and the clinical course varied from fulminating to chronic. Later, subclinical infections became well recognized. Appreciation of the nature of shunt colonization was severely hampered by both microbiologists and clinicians failing to recognize the significance of 'harmless' skin bacteria, particularly coagulase-negative staphylococci. These organisms had rarely played a role in human disease until surgical implants, of which cerebrospinal fluid shunts were almost the first, began to be used. The clinical and bacteriological features of shunt infection are described in detail in Chapters 2 and 3. The first report of an association between nephropathy and shunt colonization appeared a few years after the first reports of sepsis (Black, Challacombe and Ockenden, 1965). This condition, which became known as shunt nephritis, is discussed in Chapter 3.

2

AETIOLOGY OF SHUNT

COLONIZATION

2.1 INCIDENCE OF SHUNT COLONIZATION

Reports of the incidence of shunt colonization are difficult to analyse, as some authors report this as a percentage of patients and others report it as a percentage of operations. The latter is probably easier to grasp and is certainly more relevant to the problem. The percentages of shunt operations resulting in colonization reported in the literature is shown in Table 2.1. The figures are either quoted directly or are calculated from the authors' data. It may be seen that most publications deal with ventriculo–atrial shunts, but this is not necessarily an indication that problems of infection are greater than in ventriculoperitoneal shunts as is often thought. The ventriculo–atrial shunt was originally the most popular, partly due to the poor reputation of the early ventriculoperitoneal shunts with regard to blockage of the distal end; the first publication dealing with infection in ventriculoperitoneal shunt appeared eleven years after the first paper on ventriculo–atrial shunt infections. In addition to those data in Table 2.1, O'Brien, Parent and Davis (1979) give a combined incidence of ventriculo–atrial and venticuloperitoneal shunts of 2.7% of 778 operations. The reported incidence for ventriculo–atrial shunts ranges from 3.3 to 23% with a mean of 10.95% of 2647 operations. The incidence for ventriculoperitoneal shunts ranges from 6.2 to 22% with a mean of 12.35% of 960 operations. Bearing in mind that the data have been extracted from a number of sources and therefore are not necessarily comparable, these figures suggest that the mean reported number of infections in both ventriculo–atrial and ventriculoperitoneal shunts is similar. Differences in incidence between individual centres are likely to occur, however, and the

12

TABLE 2.1
Reported incidence of CSF shunt colonization

First author	Date	Number of patients	Number of operations	Colonization Percentage of operations VA	VP
Cohen	1961	120	120	7	
Schimke	1961	54	54	20	
Bruce	1963	300	300	6.3	
Overton	1965	48	120	3.3	
Forrest	1968	455	455	11	
Becker	1968	NS	207	7	
Luthardt	1970	183	183	9.3	
Shurtleff	1971	102	299	14	
Little	1972	74	74	14	11
Robertson	1973	297	674		6.2
Schoenbaum	1975	289	292	23	22
Bayston	1977	NS	108		10.2
Bayston	1979	NS	488	5.5	
Range, Mean				3.3–23, 10.95	6.2–22, 12.35

NS = not stated

incidence in ventriculoperitoneal shunts may be lower in centres where they are used as a primary measure than where they are used mainly in revisions.

2.2   THE NATURE AND CLASSIFICATION OF SHUNT COLONIZATION

Internal and external colonization

The organisms involved in shunt colonization are predominantly staphylococci but when *Staphylococcus aureus* is involved, the clinical picture is usually quite different from that produced by coagulase-negative staphylococci*. The illness is often more severe when due to *Staphylococcus aureus*, and there is almost always an associated infection of one of the incision sites.

* There is some confusion in the terminology of staphylococci at the time of writing. It is generally agreed that coagulase-positive strains should be referred to as *Staphylococcus aureus*, but coagulase-negative strains are often referred to as *Staphylococcus epidermidis*. The system of identification suggested by Kloos and Schleifer (1975) divides the coagulase-negative strains into several 'species', of which *Staphylococcus epidermidis* is but one. In the author's opinion, the term 'coagulase-negative staphylococcus' should be used to refer to the group of staphylococci other than *Staphylococcus aureus* until the problem is resolved.

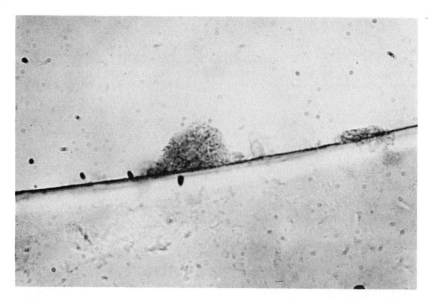

Figure 2.1 Frozen section through a shunt colonized by coagulase-negative staphylococcus. Microcolonies stained with alcian blue (magnification × 136).

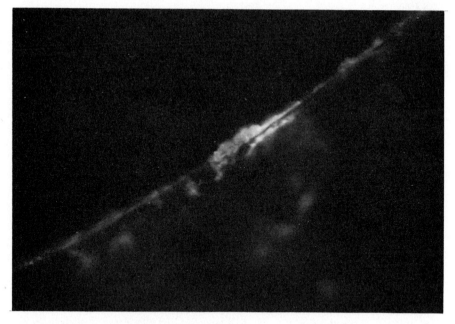

Figure 2.2 Frozen section through a shunt colonized by coagulase-negative staphylococcus. Microcolonies reacted with rabbit antibody specific for mucoid substance (slime), then stained with fluorescein-labelled antirabbit globulin (× 212).

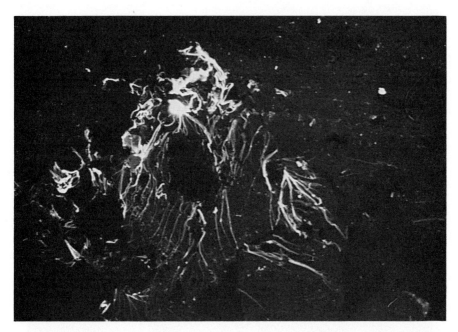

Figure 2.3 Peptone water culture of coagulase-negative staphylococcus, reacted with rabbit antibody specific for mucoid substance (slime), then stained with fluorescein-labelled antirabbit globulin (magnification × 212).

Both groups of staphylococci produce a variety of enzymes, including haemolysins, but while *Staphylococcus aureus* produces leucocidins and other antiphagocytic substances, hyaluronidases, collagenases and other proteases, coagulase-negative staphylococci appear to be unable to produce any factors which could be regarded as human toxins, with the possible exception of blepharotoxin (Valenton and Okumoto, 1973).

Certain coagulase-negative strains, however, are able to produce large amounts of extracellular slime. Using frozen sections of removed colonized shunts, we were able to show some years ago that this material probably played a major role in the adhesion of the microcolonies to the inner surfaces of the shunt, as well as in the adhesion of the cocci to each other to maintain the microcolonies (Bayston and Penny, 1972). These microcolonies, stained with alcian blue, a stain specific for carbohydrate, are shown in Figure 2.1. An antiserum to the extracellular slime was raised in rabbits, and used in fluorescent antibody stain to show the slime in the microcolonies

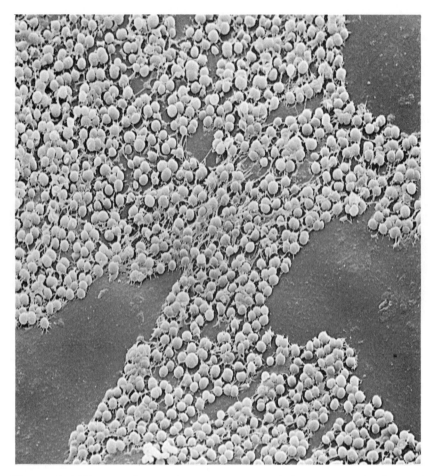

Figure 2.4 Plaque of coagulase-negative staphylococci on the luminal surface of a catheter colonized in the laboratory model. Note strands of slime extending from the bacterial surface to other cocci and to the catheter surface (magnification × 1260). SEM.

(Figure 2.2). This same antiserum was used to show slime formation by these strains in fluid culture (Figure 2.3).

The organisms which float freely in the cerebrospinal fluid in the lumen of the shunt appear to be derived from the adherent micro-colonies by shedding.

More recently, electron microscopical studies have shown the presence of extracellular slime in microcolonies in intravenous catheters (Peters, Locci and Pulverer, 1981; Christensen *et al.*, 1982)

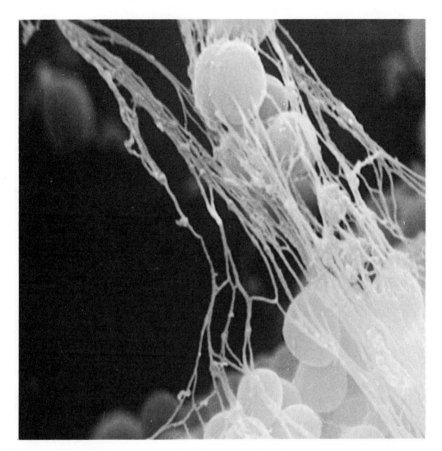

Figure 2.5 As Figure 2.4, (magnification × 1328). SEM.

and in peritoneal dialysis catheters (Marrie, Noble and Costerton, 1983).

Following the development of a reliable *in vitro* model for catheter colonization in the author's laboratory, silicone rubber shunt catheters have been successfully colonized with strains of both coagulase-negative staphylococci and *Staphylococcus aureus* (Bayston, 1984). Samples from these catheters were fixed in glutaraldehyde and examined by scanning electron microscopy. In the catheters colonized by coagulase-negative strains the microcolonies consisted of cocci embedded in a matrix of fine threads (Figures 2.4, 2.5). This material is probably analogous to that seen by the author on light microscopy of slime-producing cultures (*see* Figure 2.3). The

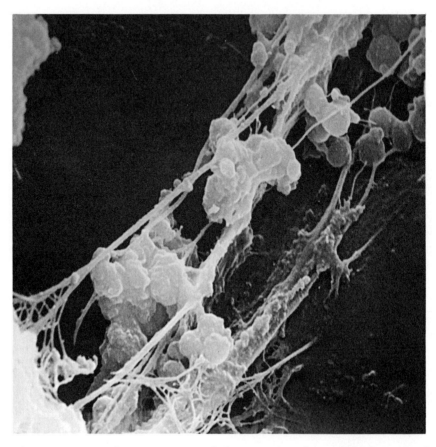

Figure 2.6 Coagulase-negative staphylococci in a colonized shunt removed from a patient (magnification × 7254). SEM. Compare with Figure 2.5. The irregular shape of the cocci is probably due to preoperative antibiotic treatment.

removed shunts from which the strains were originally isolated had also been similarly fixed and processed, and when examined by scanning electron microscopy microcolonies of identical appearance were seen (Figures 2.6, 2.7). Of course, the appearance of the slime as fine threads under these conditions is probably the result of condensation of the material during dehydration prior to the microscopy, and almost certainly does not represent the appearance of the slime *in vivo*.

Using the above model, a shunt catheter was successfully colonized with *Staphylococcus aureus* after some initial difficulty. Sections

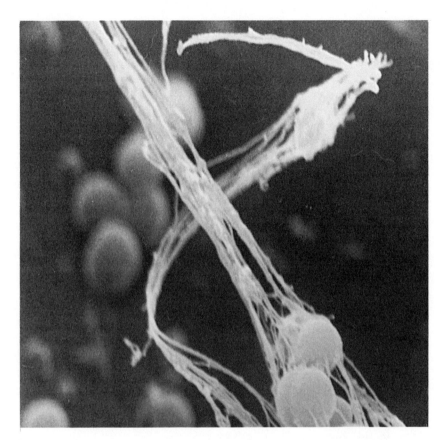

Figure 2.7 As Figure 2.6 (magnification × 1040). SEM.

of the catheter examined by light microscopy showed a thick, continuous coating of the luminal surface, but this was apparently only loosely attached and was beginning to slough off (Figure 2.8). This loose attachment was confirmed on electron microscopy (Figure 2.9). The cocci were adherent to each other but only poorly adherent to the rubber, in contrast to the tenacious attachment of coagulase-negative strains.

Other organisms such as coryneforms, which are increasing in importance in infections involving implants, may use different mechanisms of attachment, but *Corynebacterium xerosis* also appears to produce some sort of extracellular slime (Figure 2.10).

Therefore, when a shunt becomes contaminated with coagulase-negative staphylococci during insertion, those organisms on the

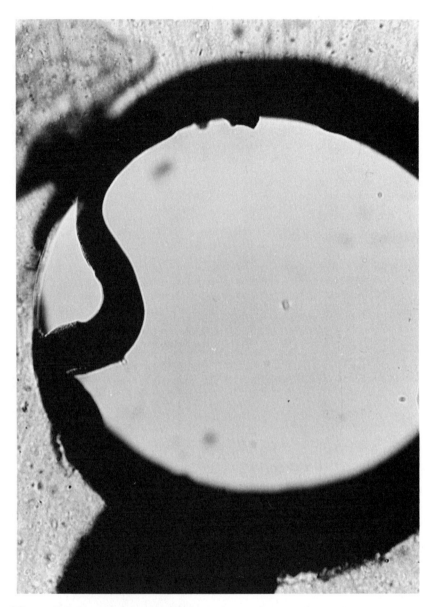

Figure 2.8 Transverse section through a catheter colonized *in vitro* in the laboratory model with *Staphylococcus aureus*. The rind of growth is loosely attached to the luminal surface.

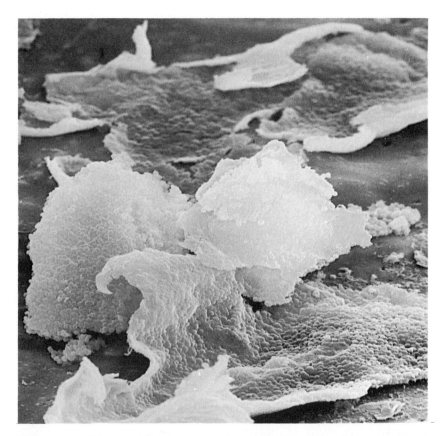

Figure 2.9 Electron microscopy of a part of the catheter shown in Figure 2.8. The organisms are attached to each other but only loosely attached to the catheter surface (magnification × 1440). SEM.

outside of the shunt will usually be engulfed and killed by the phagocytes because of this organism's lack of defensive enzymes, but those on the inside of the shunt will be protected from the host defences and may become established as microcolonies due to production of extracellular slime. This may be said to represent true colonization of the shunt. Conversely, in the cast of *Staphylococcus aureus* those inside the shunt will probably not be able to adhere efficiently to the silicone rubber, as they appear not to produce an adhesion factor, but those outside the shunt will be able to resist phagocytosis due to their toxins and will initiate a wound infection around the implanted foreign body. Occasionally, however, certain strains of *Staphylococcus aureus* do produce true, internal shunt

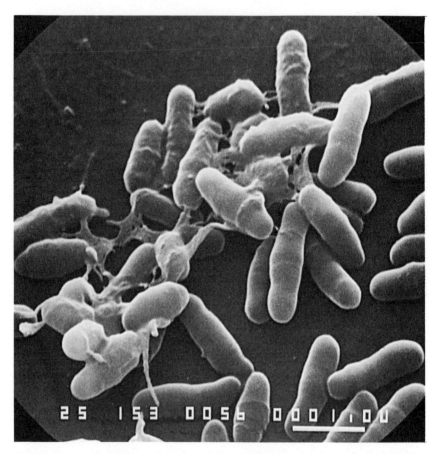

Figure 2.10 *Corynebacterium xerosis* colonizing a shunt. Note the slime extending between some of the organisms (magnification × 1395). SEM.

colonization without necessarily producing a wound infection. These strains presumably produce an adhesion factor.

Borges (1982) has shown that adherence of neutrophils and monocytes to silicone rubber shunt catheters is poor *in vitro*, and that coagulase-negative staphylococci adhering to the external surface of the catheters are not efficiently phagocytosed. This he cites as evidence for an interference with host defences by shunt material which he says could predispose to shunt infection. While this is an interesting observation, it is probably explained by the well-known resistance of silicone rubber to adherence of mammalian cells of all types. If phagocytic cells cannot adhere to the surface to which their target bacteria are attached, they will not be able to phagocytose them efficiently. This, therefore, does not imply that there is anything chemically cytotoxic about silicone rubber. It also applies only to external shunt infection, and while it may well have implications for organisms such as *Staphylococcus aureus*, the rarity of external shunt infection due to coagulase-negative staphylococci suggests that the result of this elegant study may not have general application to the majority of shunt infections. Also, Gray *et al.* (1984) have produced evidence *in vitro* which shows that the slime produced by coagulase-negative staphylococci seriously interferes with the proliferation of stimulated lymphocytes. Again, it is difficult to see how this could influence the course of an internal shunt infection, though it may well have implications for infections involving other types of implants.

From this principle shunt infections may be classified as either internal or external, the latter being basically wound infections. The vindication of this classification may be seen in numerous case reports (Schimke *et al.*, 1961; Cohen and Callaghan, 1961; Bruce *et al.*, 1963 and Luthardt, 1970). The implications for prevention, treatment and prognosis are discussed in Chapters 3, 5 and 6.

Early and late colonization

Several workers have observed that symptoms of shunt infection often appear within days or, at the most, within three or four weeks of operation, but that in some cases the patients remain symptom-free for many months or years only then to present with symptoms of 'late' or 'chronic' colonization. Schimke *et al.* (1961) first remarked upon the two groups and Shurtleff, Foltz and Christie (1971) also discussed them. In this latter series of 299 operations, all involving ventriculo–atrial shunts, 27 cases of colonization (9%) presented within four weeks of surgery. In 15 cases there was no apparent evidence of colonization until at least four weeks after operation, and one child did not become ill until six years later. In a later study (Bayston and Swinden, 1979) 9 'early' and 18 'late' cases were recorded in a series of 488 operations involving ventriculo–atrial shunts.

While early cases have been causally connected with recent shunt surgery, late cases have generally been considered to be due to occasional bacteraemias, during which staphylococci migrate up the distal catheter and through the valves, to cause shunt colonization. It was also thought that this could occur at any time after the shunt was inserted, and if the patient escaped shunt colonization at the time of surgery there was a constant risk of contracting it so long as the shunt was in position.

In an attempt to demonstrate this in the laboratory, Holt (1970) reported an experiment in which he constructed an artificial system consisting of two glass chambers, one representing the cerebral ventricular system and the other representing the right cardiac atrium, joined by tubing incorporating a Holter valve. The fluid consisted of culture medium containing a pH indicator. After introducing a strain of coagulase-negative staphylococcus into the lower chamber, and allowing fluid to flow into it by way of the valve from the upper chamber for 24 hours, the colour of the medium in the upper chamber was found to have changed, indicating a change in pH, presumably due to bacterial growth.

From this it was concluded that ascending infections from occasional bacteraemias could occur, and that the bacteria could migrate against the flow, through the slit valves into the cerebral ventricular system. However, Holt did not state whether he had compared the identity of the organism responsible for the colour change in the 'ventricular' chamber with that of those which he had introduced into the 'atrial' chamber, and chance contamination of the fluid as an explanation cannot be ruled out. Similarly, he did not state whether he had carried out the experiment once only or more than once, or whether the valve he had used was new or had been removed from a patient for some reason which could have a bearing on its function. Because of the implications of such retrograde migration of organisms up the shunt, experiments were carried out in an attempt to confirm these findings (Bayston and Spitz, 1978). Three new valves were tested using the apparatus shown in Figure 2.11, which is similar to that used by Holt.

A further series of tests on two more new valves was carried out using this system with a peristaltic pump attached so that the perfusion was pulsatile instead of constant, as pulsatile flow of cerebrospinal fluid has been demonstrated *in vivo* (du Boulay, 1966). A variety of flow rates was used, ranging from 20 ml/day to 300 ml/day. The perfusion fluid consisted of an artificial 'cerebrospinal fluid', containing 3.4 g/l sodium chloride, 0.5 g/l dextrose and 0.4 g/l of albumen. A strain of coagulase-negative staphylococcus, phage type A92/275 (27/459/275A) which had previously been isolated from a colonized shunt was used to inoculate the 'atrial' chamber. No dyes were incorporated in the system, and samples of

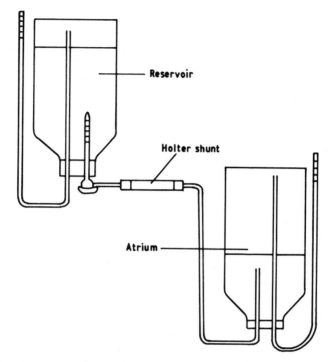

Figure 2.11 Apparatus used for testing for retrograde movement of bacteria through valves. The apparatus consists of a 'reservoir' connected to an 'atrium' by a Holter shunt.

fluid from the various components were periodically withdrawn aseptically and cultured for the presence of organisms.

In a total of 13 experiments, the sample aspirated from the 'ventricle' grew organisms on two occasions; organisms were also grown from the Rickham reservoir, from the valve chamber and from the distal catheter on these two occasions. These organisms were strains of coagulase-negative staphylococcus, but when they were typed they were found to differ from that which was originally inoculated into the 'atrium', and they were therefore considered to be contaminants, probably introduced into the system during assembly or sampling.

In all other cases the test strain was recovered from the 'atrium' and the distal catheter, but could not be cultured from elsewhere in the system. None of the valves used in the experiments allowed reflux of fluid on testing, but two of a further series of 15 Holter valves were shown to reflux when tested using back pressures of up to 400 mm of water maintained for 10 minutes. One of these allowed reflux through both valves at a back pressure of only 25 mm of water. The other allowed reflux through the distal valve only. This latter shunt had been removed because of colonization, and this had been found to involve the distal catheter and the valve chamber, but not the ventricular catheter. Four other Holter shunts removed at about the same time showed colonization confined to the distal catheter. The valves in these shunts did not allow reflux.

The obvious implications for these findings are that except in valves which allow reflux, clinical and laboratory evidence suggests that staphylococci are not capable of ascending the system past the slit valves, and therefore that ascending infections following bacteraemia due to these organisms are unlikely to occur. Further evidence discussed in Chapter 4 strongly supports these *in vitro* findings, and indicates quite clearly that 'late' infections, like 'early' infections, originate from the preceding shunt operation, but are not diagnosed promptly due to their insidious onset and vague symptomatology. There are obvious implications of this for any programme aimed at prevention.

One uncommon situation where ascending infection does occur should, however, be mentioned. Occasionally the distal catheter of a ventriculoperitoneal shunt may pierce the gut or the vagina, and become grossly contaminated with motile coliform organisms. These appear to be able to move actively up the shunt to produce intracranial gram-negative sepsis, and a mixture of organisms is often found on culturing the cerebrospinal fluid. This situation is fortunately rare, as is the similar problem of gram-negative peritonitis due to ruptured appendix in a patient with ventriculoperitoneal shunt. Here also, a mixture of coliforms and other enteric organisms, sometimes with anaerobes, ascend the shunt system.

Similarly, there is one situation in which genuine 'late' infection might occur. Here the skin over the valve, or less commonly over another part of the shunt, erodes to leave the underlying shunt visible. This may be due to poor positioning of the shunt leading to greater pressure or friction on the overlying skin, or it may be due to general ill health or to poor nutrition, or a combination of these. The eroded area inevitably becomes infected, though not necessarily due to the incursion of accepted 'pathogens', and the sepsis spreads along the interface between the catheter and the tissues until it enters the cerebrospinal fluid, the blood stream or the peritoneal cavity. This process is remarkably difficult to arrest, and when erosion occurs it almost invariably leads to shunt revision.

2.3 SOURCES OF ORGANISMS CAUSING SHUNT COLONIZATION

The majority of shunt infections are caused by staphylococci. The remainder are caused by coryneforms, streptococci of the viridans or faecal groups, aerobic Gram-negative rods and yeasts. All of these groups may be found frequently on healthy skin. The organisms found on human skin can be divided into the resident flora and the transient flora, the former being in the majority and occupying both the surface and the deeper layers, while the latter occupy usually only the surface on a temporary basis. Unfortunately, organisms such as *Pseudomonas aeruginosa* which are usually considered to be transient and not to be members of the normal resident flora, may colonize the skin for many years.

However, it is generally agreed that the resident flora of the skin usually consists mainly of coagulase-negative staphylococci, coryneforms, yeasts and propionibacteria. The numbers vary according to the sites sampled and so does the frequency with which aerobic Gram-negative rods are isolated. Typical bacterial counts from the scalp are $2.5 \times 10^5/cm^2$ aerobes, $1.3 \times 10^6/cm^2$ anaerobes, again with coagulase-negative staphylococci and propionibacteria predominating (Noble and Somerville, 1974), but the hair often contains a variety of organisms which probably reach it from the air, including *Staphylococcus aureus*, Alkaligenes and Pseudomonas (Black *et al.*, 1974). The numbers of propionibacteria vary with age, being relatively few in number in infants but increasing with the onset of puberty and the proliferation of apocrine sweat glands. The same may be said for the lipophilic coryneforms.

In those who spend long periods in hospital, and especially if they are receiving antibiotics, the skin flora is disturbed with the result that streptococci, yeasts, coliforms and *Staphylococcus aureus* are often present in large numbers.

The supposition that shunt colonization is caused by skin flora gaining access to the shunt from the patient's scalp, external ear, axilla or other areas, has been disputed from time to time by those who favour the theatre air or theatre personnel as sources. Using some of the methods of typing described later in this chapter for the strains isolated, a study of 100 operations has been carried out in order to determine the role of the patient's own skin flora in shunt infections (Bayston and Lari, 1974). Bacteriological samples were taken from the patients' skin before arrival in theatre, on arrival in theatre, and after preparation with povidone-iodine. Swabs were also taken of the external ear and anterior nares, and velvet pad cultures were taken of wounds (Holt 1966) just before closure, at the time the shunt components were being connected. Blood cultures were taken before operation and one hour, five days and ten days afterwards. The bacteria isolated were freeze-dried, and the patients were followed carefully for evidence of shunt colonization. This was eventually diagnosed in 9 patients, and the organisms isolated during those 9 operations were resuscitated and their characteristics compared to those of the organisms isolated from the colonized shunts. In 7 cases the organisms colonizing the shunts were indistinguishable from those isolated at the time of surgery from the wound, skin, ear or nose of the patient concerned. One of the 2 remaining shunts was colonized with an aerobic coryneform, the other with a viridans streptococcus. Characterization schemes for these 2 organisms were not sufficiently developed to allow comparisons to be made with isolates from the patients' anterior nares, the only site in these 2 cases from which these organisms were isolated preoperatively. Because of this, the source of the organisms in these 2 cases must remain unknown.

Strains of coagulase-negative staphylococci were isolated from 58% of wounds during operation, and in 55% of these the isolates were indistinguishable from those found on the patients' skin before entering the theatre. Where organisms not derived from the patient's skin were found, they were present in much smaller numbers. While only 4% of blood cultures taken preoperatively were positive, 29% of those taken immediately postoperatively were positive. When these organisms were typed, 16% were found to be indistinguishable from those on the patients' skin surfaces.

However, none of those patients with blood cultures positive with their own skin bacteria subsequently developed shunt colonization. Of the 9 cases of shunt colonization, only 2 had positive postoperative blood cultures and these were due to organisms not found in any previous samples. Furthermore, their shunts were not colonized with these blood culture strains, but by their own skin strains as stated above.

From this one can conclude that, when intensive typing procedures are applied to organisms isolated from such a study, the results show that cases of staphylococcal shunt colonization are usually due to organisms which are indistinguishable from those found on the skin or mucous membranes of that patient at the time of operation, and that they gain access to the shunt by way of the wound from the patient's skin during operation. This has been suggested by previous workers (Jepson, 1972). The relatively high rate of wound contamination by skin flora during surgery found in this study confirmed previous findings (Velghe, Dereymaeker and van der Voorde, 1964; Raahave, 1974).

While it is popularly believed that the air of the operating theatre, if not subjected to definite conditions of filtration and circulation, is an important source of staphylococcal wound infection, this has never been shown by direct means to be so and evidence in support of the theory has been weak.

Work by Blowers and colleagues (1955) has been cited as evidence that airborne organisms in the operating theatre can be responsible for wound infection in thoracic surgery, and that improved ventilation can improve the situation. In fact, in this investigation of frequent *Staphylococcus aureus* wound sepsis, one major cause of aerial contamination in theatre was use during operation of unsterilized blankets which had been shown to be contaminated on the wards with *Staphylococcus aureus*. Improvement of theatre ventilation was but one of a series of major changes made, one of which was to discontinue the use of ward blankets in theatre, resulting in a significant fall in the sepsis rate.

Similarly, Charnley and Eftekhar (1969) made a series of changes including the use of prophylactic antibiotics and graded improvements in theatre ventilation in total hip replacement operations and achieved a reduction in the sepsis rate from 8.7 to 1.3%. Despite the admission by the authors that they found it impossible to deduce with any degree of certainty whether 'clean' air alone had any effect, and that a new method of wound closure or antibiotic prophylaxis may have been important factors, this paper has been generally interpreted as indicating that improved theatre ventilation, preferably with laminar flow, can alone decrease sepsis rates.

It may also be noteworthy that the authors of this paper began, during the study period, to use a form of drape which was intended to isolate the skin and its cut edges from the rest of the incision. The probable importance of the cut skin edges as a source of contaminating skin flora had already been proposed by Velghe, Dereymaeker and van der Voorde (1964), and this is discussed further in Chapter 6. Moreover, it is also difficult in this sort of study to exclude the possibility that a problem such as surgical sepsis diminishes simply because it is being investigated, and all personnel become more aware of the problems and deficiencies in techniques. This is called the 'Hawthorn Effect' (Entwistle and Nisbet, 1972).

In view of the controversy surrounding the use of 'clean' air in operating theatres, a large multicentric study has been carried out in the UK under the auspices of the Medical Research Council and the Department of Health and Social Security to see whether ultra-clean air really does reduce the incidence of sepsis in operations for total hip joint replacements. The subsequent report (Lidwell *et al.*, 1982) claimed a significant reduction in sepsis in those centres where ultra-clean air was used. Unfortunately, the use of prophylactic antibiotics was not controlled (Meers, 1983a, b) and over 70% of patients received some sort of antibiotic prophylaxis during the study. Also the nature of the trial meant that changes in technique again could not be discounted as a reason for the difference, and unfortunately, no bacteriological typing procedures were included to show that those organisms causing sepsis had actually been present in the theatre air during the operation. Other orthopaedic surgeons have achieved comparable rates of sepsis while working in theatres with 'conventional' ventilation (Ring, 1974).

Shooter *et al.* (1958) could not show that airborne staphylococci were as important as those transmitted by more direct means. Our study, referred to previously (Bayston and Lari, 1974), showed that, by the use of bacteriological typing methods, at least in cerebrospinal fluid shunt infections due to coagulase-negative staphylococci, the causative organisms originated on the patient and were therefore probably introduced directly by passive movement from the skin surfaces and cut wound edges, and by gloves and instruments which had become contaminated with the patient's skin flora.

On the other hand, in circumstances where the bacterial count of the theatre air is extremely high, as in the study of Blowers *et al.* (1955), sepsis due to aerial organisms may occur but in our experience in 'conventional' theatres the number of organisms identical to those from the patient's skin found in wounds during operation far outnumber those which appear to originate elsewhere. Moreover, it is these skin organisms which cause shunt infections.

Surgical expertise and difference in technique are probably the main determining factors. In a series reported by McCarthy and

Wenzel (1977), one surgeon had a 36% shunt infection rate, while another using the same hospital facilities and in a comparable group of patients, had a rate of 5%. Similarly, in a large study by George, Leibrock and Epstein (1979) the surgeon was found to be the biggest single determining factor, with a 25-fold variance in infection rates which could be related to experience and technique.

2.4   PROCEDURES USED FOR CHARACTERIZING AND TYPING BACTERIA INVOLVED IN SHUNT INFECTIONS

A wide variety of organisms have been implicated in shunt infections (see later in this chapter) but the majority are due to the Gram-positive bacteria commonly found on the skin. These include staphylococci and the aerobic and anaerobic non-sporing Gram-positive rods, mainly corynebacteria and propionibacteria. The following discussion will be confined to these groups. With the exception of *Staphylococcus aureus*, these organisms have been long neglected by medical microbiologists because of their presumed lack of involvement in disease until relatively recently, with the result that their taxonomy and interrelationships are poorly understood.

Standard techniques are available for identification of isolates such as the aerobic Gram-negative rods, but for coagulase-negative staphylococci, *Staphylococcus aureus*, corynebacteria and propionibacteria further characterization and epidemiological typing is often desirable. In the case of *Staphylococcus aureus*, phage typing is usually all that is required, but in the case of the coagulase-negative staphylococci difficulties arise. These organisms are common skin commensals and contaminants of clinical specimens and clinically-significant isolates frequently need to be distinguished from other strains. Bacteriophage typing is available for these organisms (Verhoef, Winkler and van Boven, 1971) but in our experience this has been disappointing due to the high incidence of untypability. We have therefore resorted to the use of two other systems and one experimental system.

The coagulase-negative staphylococci can be divided into biotypes (Baird-Parker, 1963, 1965) and indeed subtypes (Holt, 1970) on the basis of biochemical tests, but these have now been superseded by the work of Kloos and Schleifer (1975) and Schleifer and Kloos (1975) who also used biochemical tests and a different scheme to divide the group into 9 'species'. Currently there are 23 species. In this author's hands the quickest and most convenient way of doing this is to use the 'API Staph.' system (API Laboratories, La Balme des Grottes, France) (Bayston *et al.*, 1983). This consists of a moulded plastic gallery of cupules each containing a freeze-dried substrate, usually with a indicator system. A standard suspension of the organism is made and added to the cupules. The gallery is then incubated overnight for 48 hours. The results are read as positive or negative reactions and a scoring system is used. A seven-digit number is produced and reference to a list of codes provided by the manufacturers will often allow the isolate to be allotted to one of Kloos and Schleifer's 'species'. The list is not, however, complete, and sometimes the 'best fit' method must be used to obtain a name for the isolate. In practice we are more interested in the seven-digit code than the name. For instance, *Staphylococcus haemolyticus* has 8 codes and *Staphylococcus epidermidis* has 32, and the use of the code itself rather than the 'species' name gives more precise identification for epidemiological purposes.

The API Staph. system was evaluated by Marples and Richardson (1982) in comparison with a modification of Baird-Parker's scheme. They found that some of the tests in the API Staph. system showed poor reproducibility, but in our experience if the period of incubation and inoculum size are controlled then reproducibility is good. They also found that the numerical code generated by the API Staph. system could be found in the index in only 30% of cases, but this is of little importance epidemiologically as the code number itself rather than the species name is used, as already stated.

The method of biotyping the coagulase-negative staphylococci currently in the eighth edition of *Bergey's Manual of Determinative Bacteriology* (1974) is Baird-Parker's modification of his own earlier method. The genus *Staphylococcus* is divided into *Staphylococcus aureus*, *Staphylococcus epidermidis* and *Staphylococcus saprophyticus*, and *Staphylococcus epidermidis* is then subdivided into four biotypes based on five biochemical tests. For epidemiological purposes, then, the Kloos and Schleifer scheme is the most useful in our hands, particularly when the API system is used.

The second system which may be used is a standardized antimicrobial susceptibility pattern, or 'sensitype' (Bayston *et al.*, 1983). The results of routine therapeutic sensitivity tests may be used for this, but it is found that its value is greatly increased if the range of drugs tested is extended beyond those considered to be of therapeutic use in

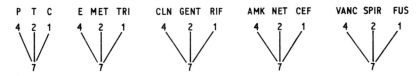

Figure 2.12 Scoring system for numerical antibiogram. P penicillin; T tetracycline; C chloramphenicol; E erythromycin; MET methicillin; TRI trimethoprim; CLN clindamycin; GENT gentamicin; RIF rifampicin; AMK amikacin; NET netilmicin; CEF cefuroxime; VANC vancomycin; SPIR spiramycin; FUS fusidic acid.

infection by these organisms. Fifteen drugs are tested in the author's laboratory by a disc diffusion method (except for methicillin) which is tested by agar incorporation at 30°C) and the results read as either sensitive or resistant with reference to controls. 'Intermediate sensitivity' or 'partial resistance' is scored as resistance. It must be emphasized that these results cannot necessarily be used to plan antimicrobial chemotherapy. The results are scored as in Figure 2.12. For example, an organism which shows resistance to penicillin, tetracycline, trimethoprim and gentamicin scores 61200.

Using the numerical biotype and sensitype a strain can be characterized by allotting a numerical code, such as 6230113/64242. This would indicate a strain of *Staphylococcus warneri* which was resistant to penicillin, tetracycline, erythromycin, gentamicin, amikacin and spiramycin. The phage type, if available, may be added to this code. Obviously, further procedures would help even more to 'fingerprint' strains, in view of their ubiquity. Research is currently in progress to assess a system based on the susceptibility of coagulasenegative staphylococci to bacteriocine-like substance produced by the aerobic Gram-negative bacilli (Bayston and Lari, 1974). Such a system has been used successfully to type strains of *Neisseria gonorrhoeae* and *N. meningitidis* (Blackwell, Young and Anderson, 1979; Blackwell and Law, 1981).

Recently, techniques based on plasmid analysis have proved successful as epidemiological tools.

Because of the renewed interest in coagulase–negative staphylococci, other techniques such as pyrolysis are currently being investigated (Magee, Hindmarch and Meechan, 1983).

In the case of corynebacteria and propionibacteria, the nomenclature is even more confused and the routine laboratory can probably do no more than attempt to identify the genus and species level, but in some cases even this may be difficult. Reference experts should be consulted where appropriate. The identification of some coryneform bacteria may involve, for example, 16Sr RNA sequencing and other chemical methods. We have until recently found it sufficient to divide these organisms into three groups: coryneforms, 'JK' coryneforms (Johnson and Kaye, 1970) and propionibacteria. The coryneform group, such as *Corynebacterium hofmannii* and *Corynebacterium xerosis*, are non-motile, catalase-positive, aerobic, non-sporing Gram-positive or Gram-variable rods, often showing a characteristic 'cuneiform' arrangement on microscopy. They usually grow readily on ordinary culture media with added blood. The 'JK' coryneforms, on the other hand, often grow very slowly on primary isolation, sometimes requiring several weeks' incubation, though in the author's hands they have typically taken 2–3 days. Biochemically, they are very inactive, with no apparent effect on carbohydrate, gelatine, urea or arginine, though they may be persuaded to produce acid from glucose and maltose if Tween 80 is added to the medium. (Jayne-Williams and Skerman, 1966). They therefore appear to be *Corynebacterium bovis* on the basis of substrate attack. The use of API 20S has been recommended for rapid identification of JK coryneforms (Kelly *et al.*, 1984). They are marked out by their comparatively slow growth on ordinary media [though a semi-selective enriched medium has been described (Wichman *et al.*, 1984)], their lack of biochemical activity and their multiple antibiotic resistance.

Propionibacteria are morphologically similar to corynebacteria on Gram film but they are anaerobic. They may become capable of growing aerobically or microaerophilically after several subcultures. *Propionibacterium acnes* produces indole, whereas the closely-related *Propionibacterium granulosum* does not. They usually grow within 2 days on anaerobic incubation but some strains take 3 days and some take much longer.

The author and his colleagues have further investigated their collection of clinically-derived coryneforms (Bayston and Higgins, 1986) and it is now considered that it is sufficient for clinical purposes to think of them as of large or small colonial type and susceptible or multiresistant to antimicrobials. The JK coryneforms, now known as *Corynebacterium jeikeium* were found to be of small colonial type but some strains were not multiresistant. Conversely, other large and small colony types which were not classified as JK were multiresistant, and it is considered that it is this feature rather than identification as *Corynebacterium jeikeium* which is important in clinical practice.

2.5   SHUNT INFECTIONS DUE TO ORGANISMS OTHER THAN STAPHYLOCOCCI

A variety of organisms which are only rarely involved in cerebro-spinal fluid shunt infections have been reported from time to time.

Coryneforms

This group of aerobic Gram-positive non-sporing bacilli live in large numbers on the skin and mucous membranes.

They have frequently been reported as causing shunt infections but they still only account for an estimated 5% or so of cases. Kaplan and Weinstein (1969) reported a case in which symptoms appeared 2 days postoperatively and the diagnosis was made within 10 days. However, as with coagulase-negative staphylococci many cases are diagnosed late, leading to some cases of immune complex nephritis. Bolton *et al.* (1975), Moss, Gary and Eissinger (1977), and O'Regan and Makker (1979) all reported cases of shunt nephritis in patients with ventriculo–atrial shunts which had last been operated upon between four and six years previously.

With the exception of the cases reported by Bolton *et al.* (1975) where the organism was *C. bovis*, causative organisms were not identified beyond the 'diphtheroid' stage, which may reflect the fact that these organisms have been neglected by microbiologists, as they have previously been considered to be harmless commensals.

The author was involved in 5 cases at Sheffield Children's Hospital, between 1973 and 1978. Four were in children with ventriculo–atrial shunts. In 1 patient the organism had been repeatedly isolated from the blood culture but misidentified as an aerobic spore-bearing bacillus (*Bacillus sp.*) and discarded as a contaminant. When the shunt was eventually removed it was found to be heavily colonized with 'diphtheroids' and the identity of the organism from the blood was then retrospectively revised. In another case the infection presented as a sinus over the Holter valve nine years after insertion. The patient was later found to have a longstanding ventriculitis with an extradural collection of caseous material which also grew co-ryneforms.

Another child was pyrexial with splenomegaly, anaemia and malaise, but negative blood cultures, for over two years before her ventriculo–atrial shunt was removed and found to be colonized with a coryneform. During this period she had undergone extensive investigations for a variety of conditions including infectious mononucleosis, Hodgkin's disease and leukaemia. Another child, after repeated revisions for shunt malfunction over 12 years, was found to have an obstruction of the distal catheter of her ventriculoperitoneal shunt. This was revised without bacteriological investigation to the ventriculo–atrial route but within one month she became pyrexial and ill and the shunt was exteriorized, at which point it was found to be colonized with a coryneform. Again, none of these organisms were fully identified.

In a more recent case in which the author was involved in London, a boy with spina bifida and hydrocephalus had a ventriculo–atrial shunt inserted. This was converted three years later to the ventriculo-peritoneal route due to suspected blockage, and it was noted that he had been intermittently pyrexial for some time. The piece of distal catheter removed at this operation grew a coryneform and one month later the shunt was again revised, still using the ventriculo-peritoneal route, due to blockage at the distal end. The organism was identified as *Corynebacterium bovis*, and labelled an atypical 'JK' organism (Johnson and Kaye, 1970). This group of corynebacteria have been involved in prosthetic valve endocarditis and cerebro-spinal fluid shunt infections and are typically relatively slow-growing and show multiple antibiotic resistance. However, our strain was doubly atypical in that it was sensitive to most antibiotics.

Since then, 4 other cases due to typical 'JK' organisms have come to our notice. In addition to vancomycin, to which all were sensitive, 3 were also sensitive to netilmicin (but not gentamicin) and rifampicin, and 1 was sensitive to rifampicin only. They were all resistant to penicillin, cefuroxime, trimethoprim, chloramphenicol and fusidic acid.

In addition, Hande *et al.* (1976) have described the case of an 11-year-old boy whose ventriculo-atrial shunt, inserted one month previously, after removal of a ventriculoperitoneal shunt, was colonized with a 'JK' coryneform. He was eventually successfully treated with intraventricular gentamicin, intravenous erythromycin and removal of the shunt

Allen and Green (1986) reported a case of a 3-year-old boy who had a ventriculo-atrial shunt inserted following removal of a medullo-blastoma. Three days postoperatively he became ill and pyrexial and the shunt was removed. A 'JK' coryneform was isolated from the aerobic blood culture bottle and from the shunt. After three days' treatment with chloramphenicol and metronidazole with external ventricular drainage (EVD) a new ventriculoperitoneal shunt was inserted. Fourteen months later the shunt protruded from the abdominal wall. The patient was well and apyrexial. Once again a 'JK' coryneform, indistinguishable from the previous strain, was isolated. The shunt was removed and the child remained well thereafter.

Propionibacterium species

These Gram-positive non-sporing rods superficially resemble co-ryneforms, but they require anaerobic conditions for primary isola-tion. Indeed, until the recent change of name they were known as *Corynebacterium parvum* or *Corynebacterium acnes*. Like some of the 'JK' coryneforms, they often grow slowly on primary isolation, in this case requiring from two to fourteen days' incubation. They are present in very large numbers in the deeper layers of the skin as part of the normal flora. Their role in the pathogenesis of acne is controversial.

Everett and co-workers (1976) reported 6 cases of cerebrospinal fluid shunt infection due to this organism. Four patients had ventri-culo–atrial shunts and 2 had ventriculoperitoneal shunts. In 1 case symptoms of infection appeared within eight hours of surgery, and in another they appeared after 18 days. In the remaining 4 cases between two and ten months elapsed before symptoms became apparent. All were pyrexial. In 3 cases these Gram-positive rods were seen in the direct Gram film of the cerebrospinal fluid while in the remaining 3 cases the results of microscopical examination were not recorded but there was cerebrospinal fluid pleocytosis and a positive culture. The time taken for the organisms to grow in anaerobic conditions varied from three to nine days.

Three cases were reported by Beeler and co-workers (1976). Two had ventriculo–atrial shunts and 1 had a ventriculoperitoneal shunt. The patients became symptomatic two weeks (the patient with the ventriculoperitoneal shunt), two months and four years after oper-ation. In the patient with the ventriculoperitoneal shunt the present-ing feature was severe generalized abdominal pain. In the patient who presented four years after surgery, and who had a ventriculo–atrial shunt, there were features of immune complex nephritis with fever, chills, gross haematuria and oedema.

Three of the 9 neurosurgical cases reported by Skinner and co-workers (1978) had cerebrospinal fluid shunts. In 1 case there were no organisms seen on microscopy but propionibacteria were isolated from removed tubing and ventricular fluid. In another the removed shunt tubing was not examined microscopically, but in the third patient Gram-positive rods were seen in the ventricular fluid at shunt removal. The shunt had been colonized for some time with coagulase-negative staphylococci and the patient was suffering from shunt nephritis.

A further case of meningitis in a child with a ventriculo–atrial shunt was reported by Brook and co-workers (1980) who also reported a fatal case of meningitis and septicaemia due to *Propionibacterium acnes* in a newborn infant without hydrocephalus.

In a study by Rekate and co-workers (1980) an apparent increase in the incidence of shunt infections due to *Propionibacterium acnes* was reported. They detected 16 cases in five years, of which 11 occurred in the last two years. The period between operation and presentation varied from one week to three years. Most patients had ventriculo-peritoneal shunts with a few having ventriculo–atrial shunts. Five patients had intraperitoneal sepsis. One patient with a ventriculo–atrial shunt which was last operated upon 18 months previously presented with hypertension and was found to have shunt nephritis. Though the authors refer to their isolates as diphtheroids, they make the point again that the organisms grow slowly and may take up to 14 days to appear on anaerobic culture.

Lim and co-workers (1980) examined all blood cerebrospinal fluid samples received in one year from neurosurgical patients for *Propionibacterium acnes*. In 275 samples of blood the organism was isolated four times, and in 455 samples of cerebrospinal fluid it was isolated 12 times. Six patients with shunts were considered to have infections due to this organism, 3 with ventriculitis, 2 with meningitis and 1 with peritonitis. The authors comment that this organism is the principal cause of meningitis after coagulase-negative staphylococci in neurosurgical patients with shunts. Again, they emphasize the importance of prolonged anaerobic cultivation if the organism is to be detected. Maniatis and Vassilouthis (1980) reported a case of infection of a craniotomy wound with *Propionibacterium acnes* after clipping of an aneurysm. The patient also had meningitis. Cohle and co-workers (1981) reported a case of secondary infection of subdural haematomas due to *Propionibacterium acnes* in a 6½-month-old infant following tapping.

An unusual case of apparently primary *Propionibacterium acnes* meningitis in a previously healthy 25-year-old man was reported by Schlesinger and Ross (1977). The patient presented with headache and left-sided tingling and weakness affecting the arm and leg, followed by nausea and photophobia. He was apyrexial. Within a few hours, left-sided motor function had returned but was replaced by right-sided weakness and facial asymmetry with slurred speech. The patient eventually recovered fully. Tests for immunological competence were normal.

The author has seen 6 cases of shunt infection due to *Propionibacterium acnes* in the past 12 months, which contrasts with only 1 in the preceding 12-month period. Cases reported to the Communicable Disease Surveillance Centre in London show that this organism is becoming more common as a cause of shunt infections, though this may be due at least partly to increased detection rates. Fortunately, all the strains examined in this laboratory have been sensitive to a wide range of antibiotics, with the exception of trimethoprim and aminoglycosides.

Listeria monocytogenes

These small Gram-positive coccobacilli are aerobic, non-sporing, motile, catalase-positive and strongly resemble corynebacteria on microscopy. They are widely distributed in nature, and have been isolated from healthy animals, sewage, decaying vegetable matter, soil and human faeces.

Heck, Hameroff and Hornick (1971) reported the case of a 65-year-old man who was a heavy drinker, and who had a shunt for normotensive hydrocephalus. He had recently complained of frontal headaches, nausea, vomiting and intermittent fever. Lumbar puncture showed a pressure of 150 mm water, xanthochromia and a white cell count of 239/mm^3, 33 of which were neutrophils. There were Gram-positive rods in the Gram film and *Listeria monocytogenes* was isolated. According to the authors the main feature of this patient's illness was dementia which resolved when the infection was controlled. *Listeria* was the cause of shunt nephritis in the case reported by Strife *et al.* (1976) of a 6-year-old girl with a ventriculo–atrial shunt for non-communicating hydrocephalus. She had been asymptomatic except for two recent episodes of painless haematuria.

The 6-year-old boy reported by Wald and McLaurin (1978) also had shunt nephritis. He had had a ventriculo–atrial shunt inserted at the age of four months. There was no history of fever, headache or vomiting, but examination revealed splenomegaly. There was no oedema or hypertension, but the boy was anaemic. Blood and ventricular fluid grew *Listeria monocytogenes*. The entire shunt was removed under high-dosage antibiotic cover. Unfortunately, immediately following insertion of a new ventriculo–atrial shunt he became pyrexial and *Listeria monocytogenes* was again isolated. The patient recovered after intraventricular methicillin therapy. It is noteworthy that this boy, like Strife's patient, presented with haematuria but was otherwise asymptomatic.

Nocardia

Infection of a ventriculo–atrial shunt with a member of the 'Rhodochrous Complex', becoming evident within two days of operation in a 6-month-old child, was reported by Boughton and Atkin (1980). Fluid aspirated from the shunt contained 75 white cells, almost all lymphocytes, and Gram-positive cocci were reported to have been seen on microscopy. The organism grew three days later.

The 'Rhodochrous Complex' consists of eight species of the genus *Nocardia* whose taxonomic positions are likely to change. They are commonly isolated from soil and have been found as aerial contaminants.

Bacillus species

These organisms are Gram-positive, aerobic, spore-bearing rods, most species of which are motile. Their spores show varying degrees of resistance to heat. They are ubiquitous, being found in soil and dust as well as various foodstuffs, and are commonly isolated from the air.

Infection due to *Bacillus cereus* in an 8-month-old infant with a ventriculoperitoneal shunt was reported by Raphael and Donoghue (1976). The child was pyrexial and vomiting, had increased tension of the anterior fontanelle and showed radiological signs of pneumonitis. The ventricular fluid showed a high white cell count but no organisms on microscopy or culture. A blood culture grew *Bacillus spp.* but this was discarded as a contaminant.

Antibiotic therapy was started nevertheless, and a second blood culture also grew *Bacillus spp.* The child remained febrile and one month later Gram-positive rods were seen in the cerebrospinal fluid. This also grew *Bacillus spp.*, as did the removed shunt. At this point, the isolates were identified as *Bacillus cereus*. There were re-evaluated and their status elevated to that of pathogen. The child recovered rapidly after shunt removal.

Cox, Sockwell and Landers (1959) reported a 4½-month-old child who developed a fever one day after insertion of a ventriculo–atrial Holter shunt. The blood and cerebrospinal fluid were reportedly sterile. For five months the child was asymptomatic but then the head circumference began to increase. The shunt was revised at the age of 1 year and was found to be blocked at the distal end. The ventricular catheter and valve were removed, leaving the atrial catheter *in situ* and four days later a new ventriculo–atrial Holter shunt was inserted on the left side. Again the child became pyrexial one day later and antibiotics were administered. A blood culture grew *Bacillus spp.* and again these were discarded as contaminants until subsequent blood culture grew the same organism. The shunt was removed, along with the old distal catheter, and these grew *Bacillus spp.* which were found to be *Bacillus subtilis*.

In the case reported by Leffert, Batist and Gidez (1970), the 5-month-old child received a ventriculo–atrial shunt, and immediately afterwards became pyrexial. The shunt was revised but the fever persisted. Blood and cerebrospinal fluid samples were reported to be growing *Bacillus spp.* and the shunt was removed. The strain was examined in detail by the authors and was found to be *Bacillus cereus*. They suggested that the phospholipase produced by this organism may induce demyelination in central nervous system infections, and this has been demonstrated in animals (Burdon, Davis and Wende, 1967).

Peptococcus

Caron *et al.* (1979) reported a 24-year-old man whose ventriculo–atrial shunt, which had been in place for eight years, was colonized with this organism. He had backache, fever and athralgia and was found to have shunt nephritis. *Peptococcus spp.*, of which there are six, are anaerobic Gram-positive cocci. They are found in the mouth, intestine and female genital tract, and have frequently been cited as causing various soft-tissue infections.

Bacteroides

These anaerobic Gram-negative rods constitute the major part of the intestinal flora and are also found in the mouth and female genital tract. Feldman (1976) reported a case due to *Bacteroides fragilis* in a 10-week-old infant who had had a myelomeningocele repaired at birth. This repair was followed by meningitis due to *Citrobacter diversus*, which led to hydrocephalus. A shunt was inserted when the infection had apparently resolved, and this was followed by the onset of persistent pyrexia and convulsions. *Bacteroides fragilis* was isolated from the blood and from the removed shunt. No brain abscess was detected.

Coliform bacteria

Numerous cases of shunt infection associated with organisms representing the aerobic Gram-negative rods from the intestinal tract have been reported. These include *Enterobacter spp.* (Lajat, Lebatard-Sartre and Guihard, 1975), and *Klebsiella spp.* (Sells, Shurtleff and Loesser, 1977; Denoya, Trevisan and Zorzopulos, 1986). Shunt infections due to coliform organisms are significantly more common in some units than in others, and this may reflect differences in practice such as the use of prophylactic antibiotics, or variations in surgical technique.

Pseudomonas

In addition to infections due to *Pseudomonas aeruginosa*, less common species have occasionally been reported. In an interesting account, Bassett, Dickson and Hunt (1973) report a child born with myelomeningocele. The lesion was swabbed with chlorhexidine before closure. A ventriculo–atrial Holter shunt was inserted six days later and povidone-iodine was used to prepare the incision sites. Low-grade pyrexia persisted for several days afterwards, but the child was discharged and remained well for 18 months. He was then admitted with flushing, pyrexia and anaemia. Blood cultures and the shunt removed at revision both grew *Pseudomonas cepacia*.

At the time the back was closed one-and-a-half years previously, the chlorhexidine had been found to be contaminated with *Pseudomonas cepacia*, and this situation had subsequently been rectified.

Isolates from the chlorhexidine and from the patient were indistinguishable serologically and biochemically, and it seems likely that the child had the organism in its cerebrospinal fluid at the time of shunt insertion.

This serves to emphasize that, even with an organism which could be expected to provoke a vigorous host reaction, the shunt becomes colonized at operation but the patient may remain well for long periods afterwards. In a case seen by the author at Sheffield Children's Hospital, *Pseudomonas fluorescens* was isolated from the lumen of a removed Holter valve. The patient had had a ventriculo–atrial shunt inserted following an air ventriculogram. One year later ventricular manometry was carried out and the cerebrospinal fluid was reported to be normal at this time. Five years later the valve was flat and the child had papilloedema. The shunt was revised and the child was well for seven months after revision but was then admitted with cervical lymphadenopathy, huge tonsils and splenomegaly. The erythrocyte sedimentation rate was raised. Antibiotics were administered and the child recovered.

Four years later, after intermittent shunt malfunction, a revision was carried out and it was then that the removed valve grew *Pseudomonas fluorescens*. Large numbers were seen in the Gram film and a heavy growth was produced on culture. The serum C-reactive protein level was raised preoperatively and the serum agglutinating antibody titre to *Pseudomonas fluorescens* rose postoperatively, a recognized phenomenon which is probably due to release of antigen during manipulation of the blocked shunt at operation. Unfortunately, unlike Bassett's case, it is not possible to say for sure when this shunt infection arose. The child made a complete recovery.

Serratia

These ubiquitous aerobic Gram-negative rods have become a more common cause of sepsis in recent years, but are still rare as a cause of shunt infection.

Four children who had Holter ventriculo–atrial shunts inserted within 16 days of each other, all of whom became infected with *Serratia marcescens*, were reported by Bruce *et al.* (1963). All became symptomatic within four days of operation, and all had positive blood cultures. Two children died. The source of the outbreak was never confirmed.

Moraxella

One case of shunt infection due to one of this group of organisms, which are members of the *Neisseriaceae*, has been reported by Lajat, Lebatard-Sartre and Guihard (1975).

Brucella

Brucella abortus is primarily an animal pathogen, being transmitted to humans who are in close contact with infected farm animals or who drink unpasteurized milk. Puri and Harvey (1981) described a child who had a ventriculo–atrial shunt inserted at the age of 4 months. At the age of 5 years he was seen again because of a two-month history of lethargy, headaches, vomiting and fever. The upper part of the valve was exposed due to skin necrosis. The child was poorly nourished and had hepatosplenomegaly and anaemia. Fluid aspirated from the shunt showed Gram-negative rods on microscopy and this, along with blood cultures, grew *Brucella abortus* type 2. Serological investigations for brucellosis showed a saline agglutination titre of 80, complement-fixation titre of 64 and an antihuman globulin agglutination titre of 1280.

The boy's father was a farmer and the family drank unpasteurized milk, though this is perhaps not the most likely route by which these organisms could have infected this patient. *Brucella abortus* is killed by gastric acid (Garrod, 1937) and the usual route of infection may well be the respiratory tract (*Lancet*, 1983). In this case infection of the erosion could also have resulted from direct contact.

Candida

This yeast-like fungus is a common inhabitor of the skin and mucous membranes. Two cases of shunt infection have been recorded by the author. One girl had a ventriculo–atrial shunt inserted at the age of 2 months, 19 days after an air ventriculogram. The operation to insert the shunt had been postponed because of suspected candidiasis of the neck creases. Three weeks later she was pyrexial, and two blood cultures grew *Candida albicans*.

The second girl had a ventriculo–atrial shunt inserted at 2 months of age. Eighteen days later the lower catheter was lengthened and routine skin swabs showed *Candida albicans* in the neck creases. The shunt continued to function poorly and was eventually removed two months later. On examination, the lower catheter was found to be colonized with *Candida albicans* and corynebacteria. The lumen of the catheter was occluded by an easily-visible plug of pseudo-mycelium which presumably was contributing significantly to the malfunction.

Mycobacteria

There are few reports of mycobacteria being involved in shunt infections. In the case reported by Gonzales, Crosby and Walker (1971) *Mycobacterium aquae* was involved. This organism, now known as *Mycobacterium gordonae*, is a scotochromogen found in tap water. The patient had a ventriculo–atrial shunt for post-haemorrhagic hydrocephalus which was later revised. One year following this revision he was admitted to hospital with coryza, cough and fever. He was found to have hepatosplenomegaly. Conventional cultures and those for tuberculosis were negative, but the liver biopsy was histologically compatible with tuberculosis and two acid-fast bacilli were seen in the specimen.

After several courses of antituberculous therapy and frequent relapses with ascites and meningitis the shunt was removed and was found to be full of acid-fast bacilli. These later proved to be *Mycobacterium aquae*.

A cautionary report of recurrent miliary tuberculosis in a patient with a ventriculo–atrial shunt was reported by Shibolet *et al.* (1979). The patient, a 21-year-old who was four months pregnant, was admitted with headache, weakness, vomiting and weight loss with a raised erythrocyte sedimentation rate. Despite negative cerebrospinal fluid findings, tuberculous meningitis was suspected and antituberculous therapy was given. The patient did not report for follow-up and the course of therapy was therefore curtailed. However, she was admitted three months later, this time to the psychiatric service, with depression and headache ten days after her child was born, and she was then transferred to neurology where she was found to have right hemiparesis and hydrocephalus. A Pudenz–Heyer ventriculo–atrial shunt was inserted and she improved slightly.

Three months later she was admitted again with fever, and chest X-ray showed diffuse miliary infiltration. Antituberculous treatment was begun and on discharge her chest film was normal. Her next admission was required four months later when she had re-appearance of miliary infiltration and a further course of antituberculous therapy was given. She was next admitted three years later with fever. Her cerebrospinal fluid was normal and no *Mycobac-terium tuberculosis* was isolated from it. A lung biopsy revealed miliary infiltration and *Mycobacterium tuberculosis* was isolated on culture of the biopsy material. Some weeks later her ventriculo–atrial shunt was found to be malfunctioning and was revised with immedi-ate neurological improvement. The patient unfortunately died from severe haemorrhage the following day. The catheter from the removed shunt grew *Mycobacterium tuberculosis*. In this case the cerebrospinal fluid was normal and the mycobacteria had apparently succeeded in colonizing the shunt, from which they seeded the lungs. While a similar case involving shunting for hydrocephalus secondary to tuberculous meningitis has not been reported, dissemination could clearly occur if the tuberculous infection had not completely resolved before shunting

However, Upadhyaya *et al.* (1983) studied 70 children with hydro-cephalus secondary to tuberculous meningitis who had ventriculo–atrial shunts inserted, and found distinct improvement in their condition but no evidence of dissemination. Bhagwati (1971) also treated 7 patients with tuberculous meningitis with ventriculo–atrial shunts during drug treatment. Despite the fact that the longest course of drug treatment before shunting in 5 of these was five weeks, and the shortest only two days, there was no evidence of miliary spread. These authors do not hesitate to recommend early shunting during the treatment of tuberculous meningitis. Suwanwela (1968), how-ever, reports cases of miliary tuberculosis after ventriculo–atrial shunting, and tuberculous peritonitis after a subarachnoid–peritoneal shunt, when shunting was carried out before the infective component had resolved.

Neisseria gonorrhoeae

A case of gonococcal meningitis and ventriculitis in a female patient with a ventriculoperitoneal shunt was reported by Noble and Cooper (1977). The patient had suffered right abdominal and flank pain with headaches and vomiting but the pain in the flank and abdomen had disappeared before admission. Four years previously she had had an Ames ventriculoperitoneal shunt inserted for hydrocephalus of un-known aetiology. On admission she was febrile with headache and neck rigidity, she also had a creamy vaginal discharge which was not submitted for culture. Fluid aspirated from the reservoir was under raised pressure (300 mm water) and had 25 white cells, 60% neutrophils. Gonococci were seen in the Gram film and were isolated on culture.

Haemophilus, meningococcus, pneumococcus

Children and adults with cerebrospinal fluid shunts are presumably equally at risk of contracting meningitis due to *Haemophilus influenzae*, *Neisseria meningitidis* and *Streptococcus pneumoniae* as the rest of the population. If they are confined in institutions, this might work to lower the incidence due to diminished exposure to the general population, or to raise it because of closer contact with fellow inmates. Nevertheless, reports of such infections in shunted patients are not common.

Two cases of meningococcal infection have appeared in the literature (Schoenbaum, Gardner and Shillito, 1975; Leggiadro, Atluru and Katz, 1984). In the first study, two cases of *Streptococcus pneumoniae* meningitis are also reported, out of a total of 289 patients. One patient had a ventriculo–atrial shunt, the other a ventriculo–ureteral shunt. The author has also seen 2 cases occurring three years apart. In the first case, and 18-month-old child with postmeningitic hydrocephalus for which a ventriculo–atrial Holter shunt was inserted was admitted after a one-day history of crying, vomiting and pyrexia. *Streptococcus pneumoniae* was isolated from both blood culture and cerebrospinal fluid. In the second case, a 3 year old with a Holter ventriculo–atrial shunt, there was a five-day history of pyrexia and vomiting. *Streptococcus pneumoniae* was isolated from blood culture and cerebrospinal fluid as well as from all parts of the shunt after removal.

Reports of cases where *Haemophilus* is involved are more frequent. Examples are: Schoenbaum, Gardner and Shillito (1975), 1 case; Raimondi, Robinson and Kuwamara (1977), 1 case; Sells, Shurtleff and Loesser (1977), 2 cases; McCullough *et al.* (1980), 1 case; Patriarca and Lauer (1980), 2 cases; Rennels and Wald (1980), 4 cases; Lerman (1981), 2 cases; Pui, Lawrence and Vanderzwagg (1981), 2 cases; and Stern, Bayston and Hayward (1988), 2 cases. Ventriculo–atrial shunts were involved in 6 cases, ventriculoperitoneal shunts in 6, with 1 each of lumbar–ureteral and lumbar–peritoneal shunts and 3 not stated. In 11 of the 12 cases where the information is given, the infections were late in onset, presenting long after any shunt surgery. In 8 of 9 cases, the patients had either preceding otitis media or a respiratory tract infection. In many cases antibiotic treatment without shunt removal was successful and these infections should probably be treated in the same manner as meningitis occurring in patients without shunts. This aspect is dealt with in greater detail in Chapter 5.

Other streptococci

Sporadic reports of shunt-associated infections due to streptococci other than *Streptococcus pneumoniae* have appeared in the literature. Perhaps the commonest, and certainly the most troublesome from a chemotherapeutic point of view, are those due to faecal streptococci or enterococci. Cases are reported in publications by Weinstein *et al.* (1977), 1 case; Villarejo (1979), 2 cases; Pui, Lawrence and Vanderzwagg (1981), 3 cases; and Males, Glaser and Shapiro (1982), 1 case.

In a case dealt with by the author, the patient was a 54-year-old diabetic with hydrocephalus secondary to a colloid cyst of the third ventricle. After shunting, he developed enterococcal ventriculitis which was eradicated only after several weeks of external drainage and systemic and intraventricular antibiotics. Few clinical details appear in the case reports in the literature, but in the author's case the organism, when first seen in the direct Gram film of cerebrospinal fluid, resembled a pneumococcus, and in the case of enterococcal meningitis reported by Ryan *et al.* (1980), in which the patient did not have a shunt, a diagnosis of pneumococcal meningitis was first made on the basis of the appearance of the organisms in the Gram film of cerebrospinal fluid.

These authors found it necessary to institute systemic and intrathecal antibiotics for a total of 33 days.

Mixed infections

Shunt infections due to a mixture of organisms usually occur in ventriculoperitoneal shunts where the distal catheter has perforated a viscus such as the gut or the vagina. Brook *et al.* (1977) described 2 cases, one with a Holter lumbar–peritoneal shunt, the other with a Heyer–Schulte ventriculoperitoneal shunt. In the first, *Escherichia coli*, alpha-haemolytic streptococci, *Bacteroides fragilis* and peptostreptococci were found in cerebrospinal fluid, and in the second *Escherichia coli* and *Bacteroides fragilis* were detected. In both cases, colonic perforation by the distal catheter was demonstrated. The fact that both these patients had had peritoneal shunt infections due to coagulase-negative staphylococci soon after surgery, which were treated non-surgically with antibiotics, is perhaps indicative of a risk factor not hitherto realized.

The author has also seen a similar case in which the patient was also treated non-surgically with antibiotics for a ventriculoperitoneal shunt infection due to a coagulase-negative staphylococcus. Three months later the patient was re-admitted, febrile and very ill. *Escherichia coli*, *Bacteroides fragilis* and *Fusobacterium* were isolated from the cerebrospinal fluid, and the lower catheter was found to have perforated the gut. A probable explanation is that, even if the staphylococcal shunt infection is eradicated, consequent adhesions and hyperplasia of local intestinal lymphoid tissue might lead more readily to perforation of the intestine. The distal end of the shunt might also be fixed by adhesions, so making it more likely to pierce viscera.

There are, of course, many other cases of shunt infection due to organisms not mentioned here, and which are not reported formally in the medical press. This can be illustrated by an inspection of the weekly Communicable Diseases Reports for UK. However, no distinction is made between true shunt infections and other central nervous system infections in patients who also have shunts, and one is left wondering whether a patient who develops ventriculitis due to *Flavobacterium*, for example, really has true shunt infection even if, as one would expect in such a case, the organism is also grown from the fluid aspirated from the shunt. From a therapeutic point of view, this situation may resemble haemophilus meningitis in the presence of a shunt, more closely than a true shunt infection (see Chapter 5).

The fact that many organisms have been reported as causes of shunt-associated infection should underline the need for microbiologists and clinicians not to dismiss any isolate as a contaminant without careful evaluation. This evaluation should include further clinical examination of the patient and the taking of another sample of cerebrospinal fluid, along with blood cultures where a ventriculo–atrial shunt is involved. Serological tests might also prove useful. Mixed Gram-negative infections, especially those in ventriculoperitoneal shunts and where anaerobic bacteria are isolated, should be considered as likely indication of visceral perforation. This possibility should also be borne in mind in any patient who has successful non-surgical treatment for an infected ventriculoperitoneal shunt.

2.6 VENTRICULITIS

Ventriculitis appears to be a frequent concomitant of shunt coloniz-ation according to some reports (Shurtleff, Foltz and Christie, 1971; Shurtleff *et al.*, 1974) while according to others it occurs rarely (Schimke *et al.*, 1961; Bruce *et al.*, 1963; Stickler *et al.*, 1968; Rames *et al.*, 1970) and in some series not at all (Callaghan, Cohen and Stewart, 1961; Cohen and Callaghan, 1961; Perrin and McLaurin, 1967; Bayston and Spitz, 1978). In a separate series of 15 cases of shunt colonization studied at Sheffield Children's Hospital, 3 chil-dren had ventriculitis. In 2 of these the infection was shown to date from the operation to insert the shunt, while in a third it was present before operation, being associated with a ventricular lavage.

The difference in incidence between centres may be due to different operative techniques, but may also be due to the different types of shunt being used.

McLaurin (1973) noted that, despite Holt's observation to the contrary, he found no clinical or laboratory evidence of retrograde extension of infection through the shunt, and we have confirmed this by both laboratory and clinical studies (Bayston and Spitz, 1978) and failed to repeat Holt's findings. Consequently, one must be aware of the possibility of obtaining a negative culture from a sample of fluid aspirated from a Rickham reservoir in a Holter shunt which may nevertheless be heavily colonized distal to the proximal slit valve. This finding is certainly not uncommon and may also occur with other proximal valves such as the Hakim.

The practice of carrying out an air ventriculogram before each shunt insertion may also lead to ventriculitis due to organisms being introduced at the time the air is injected. If the air ventriculogram is carried out within 24 hours of operation the ventriculitis may go undetected and the newly-inserted shunt often has to be removed when symptoms appear later. There are several ways of avoiding this situation. The most obvious is to use a non-invasive method of assessing ventricular size, such as ultrasound or computerized axial tomography. However, if an invasive method must be used, careful observation of the patient, including frequent temperature measure-ments, and a delay of at least 48 hours before operation are advisable. The estimation of serum C-reactive protein at daily intervals before operation may also help to detect early ventriculitis in such circum-stances (see Chapter 4).

2.7 CYSTIC BLOCKAGE IN VENTRICULOPERITONEAL SHUNTS

Colonization in ventriculo-atrial shunts does not usually lead to blockage unless *Candida albicans* is involved, when the shunt may be physically occluded by pseudomycelium. However, blockage is a very common consequence of colonization in ventriculoperitoneal shunts and is often the presenting feature. Infected cerebrospinal fluid draining from the distal end of the peritoneal catheter causes the omentum to engulf the tip of the catheter and a cyst is formed. This increases in size as it fills with fluid and eventually communicates with the fibrous sheath which usually encases the catheter. This also distends and can often be felt as a fluctuant swelling over the shunt. While the cyst can often accommodate a large amount of fluid, and the shunt may flush normally when pumped manually, neurological evidence of blockage soon develops. Such cystic blockage also occurs in the absence of infection, but there are important distinguishing features.

Between December 1974 and December 1975 the author and colleagues studied 106 operations involving ventriculoperitoneal shunts. Of these 40 were revisions undertaken because of blockage at the distal end. The Holter valve was used in all cases. Some cases of malfunction of ventriculoperitoneal shunt came to operation because of technical faults such as fracture or disconnection of the system. In others the lower catheter had been incorrectly sited or had migrated out of the peritoneal cavity. These cases, along with others involving blockage of the ventricular catheters only, were not included in the analysis.

Patients in this study who presented with signs and symptoms of raised intracranial pressure and whose Holter valve chamber emptied with difficulty on digital compression were diagnosed as having an obstruction at the peritoneal end of the system. It is important to realize, however, that flushing chambers may empty and fill normally in the presence of distal blockage. In some cases where radio-opaque contrast material was injected into the system, a collection of contrast around the tip of the distal catheter indicated the presence of a cyst. In these cases contrast material could often be seen refluxing around the outside of the catheter (Figure 2.13).

In all of the 39 cases included in the study, blockage of the peritoneal catheter was confirmed at operation. The cause of the

TABLE 2.2

Features of 11 cases of VP shunt colonization

Pyrexia	8
Abdominal pain	5
Neutrophilia	3
Blockage distal end	11

blockage was found to be local peritoneal or omental adhesions and cyst formation (Figure 2.14). Colonization of the ventriculoperitoneal shunt was diagnosed in 11 of these cases. In addition to the signs and symptoms of blockage most of these patients were pyrexial. Abdominal pain featured in 5 (Table 2.2). Only 3 patients had positive blood culture, and only in these patients did the serum antibody titre to coagulase-negative staphylococci rise (see Chapter 3). In the author's subsequent experience, a positive blood culture is rare in patients with ventriculoperitoneal shunt colonization.

The time elapsing between operation and presentation was then examined. Twenty-four cases presented more than one year after surgery but the 11 colonized cases all presented within two months of operation (Figure 2.15).

Most patients in this study were followed-up serologically as a matter of course (see Chapter 4). The serological results revealed that, in 9 of the 11 colonized cases, the serum C-reactive protein (CRP) was raised whereas in those whose blockage was not infective in origin it was normal. In the 2 remaining colonized cases the test was not carried out.

Evidence in the literature also supports the observation that in patients with ventriculoperitoneal shunts, blockage at the distal end, if associated with infection, presents within a few months of operation. Fischer and Shillito (1969) reported 3 cases of intraperitoneal cyst in patients with ventriculoperitoneal shunts. Two had had shunt infections just prior to the insertion of the present shunt. In one of these cases, however, the infection may have been eradicated by antibiotics and shunt revision, as the cystic blockage occurred 21 months afterwards and no organisms were found in the cyst fluid. Similarly, Grosfeld *et al.* (1974) reported 3 cases of cystic blockage, 1 of which occurred eight months postoperatively, with no evidence of infection. Of the remaining 2 cases, 1 presented two months, the other three months after operation. Both had fever and abdominal

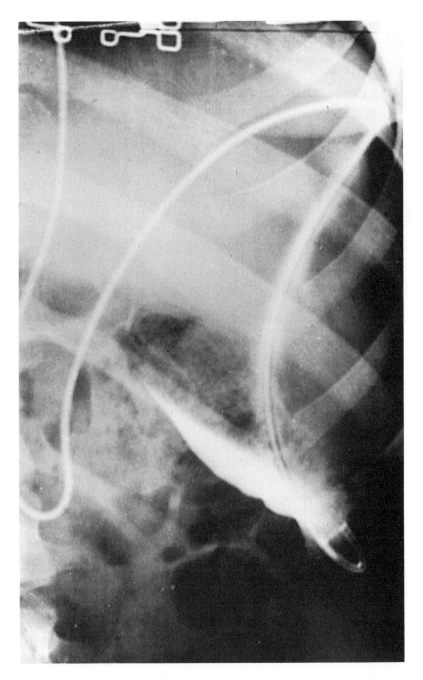

Figure 2.13 Contrast radiograph of the distal portion of a blocked ventriculoperitoneal shunt, showing contrast medium failing to disperse and beginning to reflux up the outside of the shunt. (By courtesy of Professor L. Spitz.)

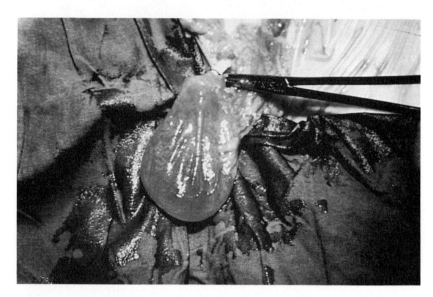

Figure 2.14 Fluid-filled cyst attached to the distal end of a ventriculoperitoneal shunt. (By courtesy of Professor R. B. Zachary.)

pain. *Staphylococcus aureus* was isolated from the fluid in one cyst but no organism was isolated from the other case despite the finding of purulent fluid in the cyst. Parry, Schumaker and Llewellyn (1975) reported 4 cases with cysts presenting one week, 12 days, one month and one month respectively after operation. One was due to *Staphylococcus aureus* but the other 3 were on high-dose antibiotics at the time and no organisms were isolated. The authors were of the opinion that all 4 were infected. The patient reported by Latchaw and Hahn (1981) presented with abdominal pain and fever one month postoperatively. The distal catheter was resited within the abdomen and no organisms were found in the cyst. Six months later the patient again had fever and chills and a septic wound from which were grown corynebacteria, *Escherichia coli*, klebsiella, clostridia, enterococci and enterobacteria. The ventricular fluid also persistently grew the latter two organisms. It is possible that the collection of faecal organisms was derived from a perforation of the intestine by the distal catheter (Wilson and Pertan, 1966; Brook *et al.*, 1977) following the earlier shunt infection, but the shunt was exteriorized and it is also possible that the persistent finding of organisms in the cerebrospinal fluid cultured was due to their colonizing and persisting in the drainage tube. Rodgers, Vries and Talbert (1978) reported

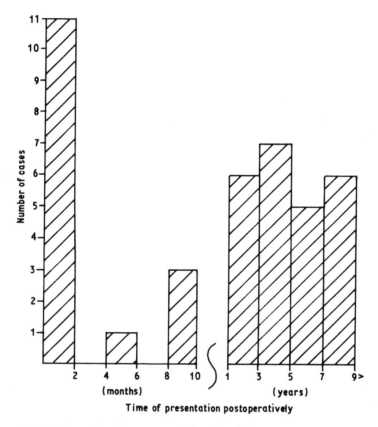

Figure 2.15 Time of presentation of distal end obstruction in 39 cases. All had ventriculoperitoneal shunts. Only those 11 cases presenting within 2 months of operation were found to be infected.

4 cases of distal blockage in ventriculoperitoneal shunts. All presented within three months of operation. Using a laparoscope, cysts could be seen in 3 cases, and omental adhesions in the fourth. Two were shown to be infected, with Candida and coagulase-negative staphylococcus respectively, and in 2 no organisms were found.

The association between shunt infection and cystic blockage in ventriculoperitoneal shunts has not always been appreciated, and evidence of infection has not always been sought. Of 49 ventriculoperitoneal shunts revised by Ignelzi and Kirsch (1975), 37 were blocked by omental or peritoneal adhesions, and about one-fifth presented within one month of operation. Most of Keucher and Mealey's (1979) cases with distal blockage presented within four months of the operation but in both these papers sepsis as a cause was not looked for. Little, Rhoton and Mellinger (1972) and Robertson, Maraqa and Jennett (1973) reported between them 76 revisions for distal blockage of ventriculoperitoneal shunts, and found only one cyst and no peritonitis. Ivan, Choo and Ventureyra (1980), reporting 97 ventriculoperitoneal shunt revisions, found 10 cases with cysts or adhesions. The reasons for the low incidence of cysts and adhesions reported by some workers may be that the abdomen was not fully explored during revision, and radiological examination, particularly using contrast material, was not done. Fischer and Shillito (1969) carried out exploratory laparotomy on their patients, as did Parry, Schumaker and Llewellyn (1975). Grosfeld et al. (1974) used radiological contrast studies to detect cysts, and Latchaw and Hahn (1981) used gallium scans and computerized tomography.

In order to avoid delay in treatment and successive operations to free adhesions, it is important to diagnose the infective component of cystic blockage preoperatively. Blockage of the distal end of a ventriculoperitoneal shunt should be suspected as being due to colonization if symptoms appear within two to three months of previous surgery, and if the serum C-reactive protein is raised. The value of this test in the diagnosis of shunt colonization must be emphasized. Where the patient is receiving antibiotics, this period may be lengthened considerably, and the serum C-reactive protein may be normal due to suppression of intraperitoneal inflammation, but this rarely remains so for long. It is also worth noting that in shunts using the Holter valve, colonization may be confined to the distal catheter only and a bacteriologically negative aspiration from the valve chamber or reservoir may mislead one into believing that colonization is not present.

2.8 SUMMARY

1. Wide differences in the incidence of shunt colonization occur between centres and between operators;
2. Overall there is little difference between infection rates in ventriculo–atrial and ventriculoperitoneal shunts, though again large differences may be experienced in individual centres, possibly due to unfamiliarity with one or other route;
3. Shunt colonization can be classified as internal, which is true

colonization of the shunt and is usually due to coagulase-negative staphylococci, or external, which is really a soft-tissue infection enhanced by the foreign material, and is rarely caused by co-agulase-negative staphylococci;

4. 'Early' and 'late' infections do not exist as separate aetiological entities. 'Late' infections have the same cause as 'early' ones but take longer to become obvious;
5. In the vast majority of cases, the organisms causing shunt colonization are derived from the patient's skin during operation;
6. Because the organisms causing most cases of shunt colonization are in most other circumstances only rarely involved in infective processes, little is known of their bacteriological characteristics and epidemiological typing schemes are rudimentary or lacking;
7. A large number of organisms has been reported as causing shunt infections and none, however bizarre or unusual, should be dismissed as due to contamination until thoroughly investigated;
8. Early cystic blockage in ventriculoperitoneal shunts is often secondary to shunt colonization.

3

DIAGNOSIS OF

SHUNT INFECTION

3.1 CLINICAL FEATURES OF SHUNT
COLONIZATION

The clinical features of shunt colonization vary with the organism involved, whether the route of shunting is ventriculoperitoneal or ventriculo–atrial, and in ventriculo–atrial shunts whether the condition is 'early' or 'late' (see Chapter 2).

When *Staphylococcus aureus* is the infecting organism the onset is generally earlier in all types of shunts, with external colonization giving rise to erythema over the shunt track and delayed healing or suppuration at one or more incision sites. In some cases the more prominent parts of the shunt, usually under the scalp, may be exposed. Systemic symptoms are usually, but by no means always, present. The blood leucocyte count may be raised, and the blood culture is often positive. Chills, fever and rigors may occur. C-reactive protein is present in the serum in increased amounts and the titre of antibody to coagulase-negative staphylococcus does not usually rise, but a rising titre of antibody to the infecting strain of *Staphylococcus aureus*, and sometimes to its alpha-toxin, can be demonstrated. However, these tests are often superfluous and the diagnosis of infected shunt with a blood and cerebrospinal fluid culture positive for *Staphylococcus aureus* should signal the need for prompt removal of the device.

A similar picture is sometimes found when the infecting organism is a member of the coliform group or a related species, but there is often more marked evidence of systemic infection, sometimes progressing to septic shock and disseminated intravascular coagulation

TABLE 3.1
Clinical features of shunt colonization

Ventriculo–atrial	Ventriculoperitoneal
Intermittent fever	Intermittent fever
Anorexia	Anorexia
Anaemia	Abdominal pain or discomfort
Lassitude	Cystic swelling over distal end of shunt
Splenomegaly	Later swelling around catheter track
Transient rashes	Erythema over catheter track
Arthralgia	Headache, vomiting, visual disturbances
Present weeks, months or years after operation	Present within 2–3 months of operation
Shunt malfunction is not usually causally related	Shunt malfunction is usual and may be the presenting feature

(DIC). Septic shock with DIC can also occur in *Staphylococcus aureus* infections, and the prognosis is poor in such cases. However, serious illness is not the invariable consequence of shunt infection due to Gram-negative organisms, and their presence may go unsuspected for long periods.

A girl whose Holter ventriculo–atrial shunt was revised in Sheffield Children's Hospital because of blockage, had mild headaches for some time and had developed papilloedema. The shunt was examined by the author after removal and large numbers of *Pseudomonas fluorescens* were found on microscopy and culture of fluid taken from inside the valve pumping chamber. The infection was not suspected at operation and a new shunt was inserted, with no subsequent ill-effects or recurrence of infection. The child had a serum agglutinating antibody titre to the pseudomonas of 20 which rose to 320 postoperatively. A rise in antibody titre following revision of a blocked shunt which is also colonized is not uncommon, and is presumably due to release of antigen into the circulation during operation.

The child had undergone ventricular manometry ten years previously, and five years previously had been admitted with papilloedema due to shunt malfunction, when a ventricular tap was carried out. Six months later, that is four years before the shunt was revised, she was admitted with a fever and was found to have cervical adenopathy, grossly enlarged tonsils, splenomegaly and an erythro-cyte sedimentation rate of 40 mm in half an hour. At this stage, shunt colonization was not suspected and she was treated symptom-atically.

Patients whose ventriculo–atrial shunts are colonized with co-agulase-negative staphylococci may remain almost asymptomatic for long periods, or they may become ill within a few days of operation. This may be due to differences in host response, or in the potential of the infecting strain to produce toxic or immunogenic factors as yet unidentified. Experimental evidence suggests that the flow rate through the shunt, governing the supply of nutrients to the organisms, might be an important factor. In some patients who present years after operation the shunt is found to be malfunc-tioning, and it may actually be the consequences of malfunction, rather than infection, which first attract medical attention. Presum-ably, in these cases the lack of symptoms can be explained by the organism being incarcerated in the shunt. When a careful history is taken in such cases, and particularly where blood culture or serologi-cal tests have been carried out at intervals since operation, evidence can often be found of intermittent, if infrequent, bouts of bac-teraemia.

Ventriculo–atrial shunt infection

The features of ventriculo–atrial shunt infection with coagulase-negative staphylococci are intermittent fever, sometimes with rigors, splenomegaly, anorexia and anaemia. If the condition is allowed to persist, evidence of early immune complex disease may appear, such as intermittent painful, swollen joints and a morbilliform rash which may appear fleetingly, only to disappear again within an hour or so. Later, haematuria, proteinuria, cylindruria, loin pain and oedema indicate the onset of shunt nephritis. Another complication of the use of ventriculo–atrial shunts is thrombus formation. Emery and Hilton (1961) found, in a series of 15 necropsies, that thrombus formation in the superior vena cava, the jugular and other tributary veins was common. Thirteen cases showed pulmonary emboli, and at least 5 of these were described as septic or suppurative, although the infecting organisms were not given. These findings were later confirmed by Erdohazi, Eckstein and Crome (1966), though the problem appears to have decreased possibly due to the use of better biomaterials or to the decreased incidence of *Staphylococcus aureus* shunt infections.

Ventriculoperitoneal shunt infection

The features of ventriculoperitoneal shunt infection are somewhat different. The patient may present with signs of raised intracranial pressure rather than with those of sepsis. This is often due to blockage of the distal catheter by a cyst (see Chapter 2) which may be palpable, and may extend up the catheter track. Where this occurs, erythema may be present over the catheter. The coagulase-negative staphylococcus is usually the causative organism. Signs of generalized sepsis may be absent and blood cultures are usually negative, so that without serological tests, the infective component may be missed. This will usually have serious consequences, as illustrated by the case of a 2-month-old girl with spina bifida and hydrocephalus. She had ventriculitis due to coagulase-negative staphylococci soon after repair of her myelomeningocele, and this cleared clinically and bacteriologically on antibiotic treatment. Three weeks after stopping this treatment she was still well, and had a Holter ventriculoperitoneal shunt inserted. Immediately postoperatively she became pyrexial and was given gentamicin intramuscularly for one week. She became apyrexial and was generally well. Her serological results remained normal, including the serum C-reactive protein level, for the following three weeks, but no more tests were carried out until the child attended a routine outpatient clinic three months later. The child was well although her parents said she had appeared rather 'hot' a few days before. There was no evidence of sepsis or shunt malfunction. Serology showed a C-reactive protein level of 3+ and an antibody titre to coagulase-negative staphylococcus of 1280 (normal for this age 20). The high antibody titre is unusual in a patient with a colonized ventriculoperitoneal shunt, but this and the C-reactive protein level made this diagnosis possible. However, at the time insufficient experience of the C-reactive protein test had been gained, and in view of the child's general good health it was decided to take no immediate action but to see her again as an outpatient in the near future. Unfortunately she was brought in dead to the casualty department before she could be seen again. At necropsy there was a peritoneal cyst with peritonitis and peritoneal abscesses and a coagulase-negative staphylococcus was isolated from these sites and from the fluid in the lower catheter, but not from the more proximal parts of the shunt. The organism had the same characteristics as that which had previously caused the ventriculitis following back closure. It is conceivable that had the experience with shunt serology been greater, so that the significance of the results had been appreciated, prompter action might have been taken. The diagnosis of colonized ventriculoperitoneal shunt is difficult to make if only the distal catheter is involved and serological testing is essential.

Ventriculoperitoneal shunt infection can also simulate acute abdomen, as described in 19 cases by Reynolds, Sherman and Malone (1983). Three had laparotomy for suspected appendicitis, and 1 had an unnecessary intestinal resection. While bacteriological details are not given, 65% grew Gram-positive organisms and 23% grew Gram-negative rods.

Where *Staphylococcus aureus* is involved, the abdominal wound often suppurates and the catheter tip may protrude, although this may occur with sepsis due to other organisms, and sometimes in the absence of sepsis. The erythema over the catheter is usually greater than that seen with coagulase-negative staphylococci and there are often signs of generalized toxaemia with pyrexia, raised blood leucocyte count and positive blood culture.

Shunt nephritis has not been reported in patients with ventriculoperitoneal shunts.

3.2   SHUNT NEPHRITIS

Four years after the first report of ventriculo–atrial shunt colonization (Callaghan, Cohen and Stewart, 1961) 2 cases of nephrotic syndrome were reported in children whose shunts were colonized with coagulase-negative staphylococci (Black, Challacombe and Ockenden, 1965). The shunts were removed and the nephrotic syndrome subsided, leading the authors to suspect a causal association. Since then numerous other reports of nephropathy in association with ventriculo–atrial shunt colonization have appeared in the literature (Holland, 1967; Stickler *et al.*, 1968; Rames *et al.*, 1970; Kaufman and McIntosh, 1971; Moncrieff *et al.*, 1973; von Moltz and Doswald, 1976; Bayston and Swinden, 1979) and the subject has been reviewed (Futrakul, Suprapathana and Campbell, 1970). The term 'shunt nephritis' was first used by Stauffer (1970) to describe this condition.

In his original report Black noted that IgG and complement were demonstrated in renal biopsy material from 1 case, and this has been confirmed many times by others using both immunofluorescence and electron microscopy. Shunt nephritis is now known to be due to the formation of immune complexes and their deposition on the basement membranes of the glomeruli. In this respect the pathogenesis of the glomerular lesions is similar to that of glomerulonephritis following infections with Lancefield Group A beta-haemolytic streptococci (Michael *et al.*, 1966). Baehr and Hande (1920) described a similar lesion in patients with subacute bacterial endocarditis due to viridans streptococci, and Boulton-Jones *et al.* (1974) also reported glomerulonephritis in patients with endocarditis due to coagulase-negative staphylococci. No evidence of septic embolization, such as is seen with *Staphylococcus aureus*, was found in their patients and the lesions were found to be associated with immune complex disease.

While coagulase-negative staphylococci are almost always the organisms associated with shunt nephritis, the condition has been reported as a complication of shunt infections due to propionibacterium (Beeler *et al.*, 1976) and another case involving coryneform organisms was encountered in Sheffield Children's Hospital in 1976 in a 7-year-old girl who presented with splenomegaly and pyrexia and later developed haematuria.

In a recent study of 11 cases of shunt nephritis due to coagulase-negative staphylococci (Bayston and Swinden, 1979) only 1 case did not have a recorded fever. All were anaemic and 6 had splenomegaly. Three had arthralgia and 5 had recurrent transient rashes before the onset of nephritis, suggesting that the immune complex disease does not affect only the glomerular basement membranes, and that these may become involved relatively late in the disease. This is further suggested by the length of time between shunt surgery, the assumed time of onset of shunt infection (see Chapters 2 and 4), and diagnosis of shunt nephritis which ranged from 21 months to ten years in this study (Table 3.2).

Because serological diagnostic methods were used, many patients showed only laboratory evidence of immune complex glomerulonephritis, and only 2 patients were oedematous. All had proven ventriculo–atrial shunt colonization, with elevated serum antibody titres to coagulase-negative staphylococcus ranging from 1280 to 10 240. Serum C-reactive protein level in the 9 patients tested was raised, and all patients had depressed serum complement levels. After removal of the shunt, antibody titres and C-reactive protein levels returned to normal and urinary abnormalities disappeared in 9 patients except for 1 case where albuminuria persisted. Of the

TABLE 3.2

Main features of 11 cases of shunt nephritis

Case no.	Fever	Anaemia	Splenomegaly	Arthralgia	Rash	Oedema	Haematuria	Albuminuria	Cylinduria	Plasma urea (mmol/l)†
1	+	+	+	−	−	+	+	+	+	4.2
2	+	+	−	−	−	−	+*	+	+	6.6
3	+	+	−	−	−	−	+*	−	−	5.4
4	+	+	+	+	+	−	+	+	−	5.4
5	+	+	+	+	−	−	+	+	+	6.7
6	+	+	−	−	+	−	+	+	−	6.5
7	+	+	+	+	+	+	+	+	+	6.0
8	+	+	+	−	+	−	+	+	+	14.2
9	+	+	+	−	+	−	+	−	+	8.64
10	+	+	−	−	−	−	+	−	−	ND
11	−	+	−	−	−	−	+	+	−	7.1

* Microscopic haematuria but more than 20 RBC/HPF.
† Normal range for plasma urea, 2.7 – 6.3 mmol/l.
ND Not done.

remaining 2 patients, 1 died shortly after operation and the other returned to her country of origin and was lost to follow-up.

The above study (Bayston and Swinden, 1979) involved 488 children who had had insertion or revision of a ventriculo–atrial shunt. Eighteen cases of 'late' shunt colonization were detected using serological methods, but only 1 of these (case 11) had been followed-up under a serological surveillance programme (see Chapter 4). The patient, a six-month-old girl, had undergone multiple shunt revisions because of blockage and infection. Routine serological testing ten days after the most recent insertion of a ventriculo–atrial shunt showed that the new shunt was colonized with coagulase-negative staphylococci, and this was confirmed by blood cultures. Because of technical problems involved in further revisions and because she was asymptomatic she was given oral cloxacillin and sent home to be observed frequently as an outpatient. She remained asymptomatic but became anaemic and the antibody titre to coagulase-negative staphylococcus continued to rise.

Fourteen months after diagnosis the titre had risen to more than 10 240, the serum C-reactive protein test was positive and the serum complement level was depressed. Shunt nephritis was suspected, but there was still no clinical evidence of this condition. Three months later the serum findings were essentially unchanged, but she had developed haematuria and a raised plasma urea level and her anaemia had worsened. Surgical intervention was now reconsidered, and a carefully planned operation involving removal of the colonized shunt and insertion of a ventriculoperitoneal shunt on the opposite side was successful. Following this the laboratory signs returned to normal.

The remaining 17 patients had not had any serological screening following shunt surgery, until that which was done to confirm the diagnosis. When Case 11 is excluded, the minimum length of time from operation to diagnosis is three years.

This association between delay in diagnosis of ventriculo–atrial shunt infection and development of shunt nephritis is very important. It emphasizes the fact that immune complex nephritis is entirely preventable by prompt diagnosis, and this can easily be made using serological surveillance (see Chapter 4).

The development of shunt nephritis in patients with colonized ventriculoperitoneal shunts has not been recorded, and the author has not seen this happen. This is not unexpected if it is considered that for an immune complex disease such as shunt nephritis to develop there must be high levels of circulating antibody and antigen, and we know that in the case of ventriculoperitoneal shunt colonization with coagulase-negative staphylococci the serum antibody titre does not usually rise and the blood culture is almost always negative. However, the author has encountered a patient whose shunt nephritis developed during a long-standing ventriculo–atrial shunt infection with coagulase-negative staphylococci. The shunt system was revised to ventriculoperitoneal with recurrence of infection and a consequent series of revisions, during which time the shunt nephritis remained active with no decrease in circulating antibody, and resolved only when the ventriculoperitoneal shunt infection was successfully treated.

3.3   OTHER MANIFESTATIONS OF IMMUNE COMPLEX DISEASE

In addition to shunt nephritis, other manifestations of immune complex disease have been reported. As already mentioned, a neglected feature of many cases of shunt nephritis is arthralgia. Pinals and Tunnessen (1977) reported a case in which juvenile rheumatoid arthritis was diagnosed following intermittent leg pain and swollen knees. This diagnosis was made five years after the insertion of a subdural–jugular shunt but the patient had had arthralgia for over a year. He had a positive rheumatoid factor titre, anaemia, raised erythrocyte sedimentation rate, depressed serum complement level and evidence of shunt nephritis on renal biopsy. The shunt, which was infected with coagulase-negative staphylococci was removed with subsequent rapid recovery. In the author's experience, arthralgia appears earlier than evidence of nephritis, but this may be because the former is more obvious to the patient, and nephritis is often not diagnosed at least until haematuria and back pain appear.

The rash is an equally neglected feature, and is also probably due to immune complexes. The author was involved in a case of a doctor who had an aneurysm clipped and then developed hydrocephalus for which a shunt was inserted. Approximately one year later he developed a haemorrhagic ulcer on the left ankle which was thought at the time to be a 'penicillin rash'. A few weeks later he sought dermatological advice because of further haemorrhagic lesions. These were biopsied and the section showed fibrinoid necrosis of dermal vessels, some which were thrombosed, with fragmentation of white cells and extravasation of red cells. The appearances were considered to be those of necrotizing vasculitis. This was thought to be associated with septicaemia and the probable connection between this possibility and the presence of ventriculo–atrial shunt was realized. Blood cultures were negative but the antibody titre to coagulase-negative staphylococcus was 1280 and the serum complement was low. The shunt was aspirated and was found to be colonized with coagulase-negative staphylococci. After antibiotics and shunt removal the patient recovered and the rash resolved.

Pneumonopathy has been reported (Macheret *et al.*, 1974) in one patient. Dyspnoea appeared three weeks after insertion of a first ventriculo–atrial shunt, and worsened over the following nine months. On examination at this time he was afebrile. There was a rash on the legs and forearms. Laboratory examination revealed anaemia, raised IgG, and normal complement levels. Leucocytes, erythrocytes, casts and protein were present in the urine. Six blood cultures grew coagulase-negative staphylococci. Renal biopsy showed deposits of complement and immunoglobulin on the glomerular basement membranes. Lung biopsy showed focal alveolitis and arteritis with immunoglobulin and complement deposits. Following removal of the infected shunt, the patient's condition improved remarkably, with disappearance of dyspnoea and rash.

This case is unusual in several aspects, not least being the extremely early onset and the pulmonary involvement. One is led to suspect that this particular patient may have had an underlying immunological anomaly such as Goodpasture's syndrome. However, it is also likely that, if biopsy material from various sites in patients with colonized ventriculo–atrial shunts were examined immunologically, more evidence of involvement of skin, lungs, synovial membranes and other tissues as well as the renal glomeruli would probably come to light. While these data would be interesting from an academic standpoint, the taking of biopsies, including renal biopsies for the diagnosis of shunt nephritis, is not justifiable as the prime diagnosis is that of infected shunt, towards which treatment should be directed. Renal involvement can be implied by clinical examination, estimation of serum complement levels and examination of the urine.

3.4   LABORATORY PROCEDURES

Blood culture

The finding of a positive blood culture in a patient with ventriculo-peritoneal shunt which is colonized with coagulase-negative staphylococci is very uncommon, although where *Staphylococcus aureus* or coliform organisms are involved these may often be recovered by blood culture.

Positive blood culture is a more common finding in patients with colonized ventriculo–atrial shunts, but repeatedly negative blood cultures in the presence of proven ventriculo–atrial shunt colonization are not unusual.

Contamination is also a problem. This may arise from the patient's skin, from the phlebotomist's fingers, or during laboratory manipulation. Common blood-culture contaminants therefore, are coagulase-negative staphylococci, coryneforms, viridans and faecal streptococci, aerobic spore-bearing bacilli and occasionally coliform organisms and clostridia, especially when blood is taken from babies or by femoral puncture. Unfortunately, one can never lightly dismiss such organisms as contaminants as most have been reported as causing shunt colonization. This dilemma can perhaps best be resolved by including serological tests in the diagnostic armamentarium (see Chapter 4).

The proper technique of drawing blood for culture is well known and to describe it here in detail would be superfluous. However, in view of the problem of contamination, special attention should be paid to preparation of the patient's skin and to the phlebotomist's fingers. A commercially-available pad soaked in isopropyl alcohol (e.g. Mediswab) is sufficient for this, and a non-volatile antiseptic such as chlorhexidine or iodine should never be used as this may itself contaminate the blood culture and inhibit bacterial growth. Another method of drawing blood for culture is that described by Holt (1966) using capillary blood from the heel or finger. In the author's experience when this is carried out properly, the contamination rate does not exceed that of venous blood cultures, but there is some doubt about the positivity rate, as organisms such as coagulase-negative staphylococci are rapidly phagocytosed and most may have been engulfed and killed before reaching the capillary bed of the extremities.

While no time should be wasted in achieving a result, systematic subculture of blood cultures from patients with shunts is not advisable as it increases the risk of contamination. With experience one can determine signs of growth by careful daily visual inspection, unless an opaque medium is used. Alternatively, a radiometric system (Bactec) can be used. It must be emphasized that under no circumstances should any isolate from a blood culture from such a patient be assumed to be a contaminant. Antibiotic sensitivities should be carried out on all isolates, even if only for purposes of comparison with previous or subsequent isolates. It should be remembered that a number of tragedies have been due to assumption of microbiologists and clinicians that unusual or 'commensal' organisms isolated from the blood of patients with shunts are contaminants.

In the author's experience, multiple blood culture does not necessarily overcome the problems of negativity or contamination and may even compound them, in that a blood culture which is positive for one organism (due to contamination) may be followed by one which is positive for a different organism or a mixture of organisms (also due to contamination). Also, it is not unknown for consecutive blood cultures to be contaminated by the same strain. However, isolation of the same strain from two or three consecutive well-taken blood cultures is very suggestive of ventriculo–atrial shunt colonization.

In the case of suspected ventriculo–atrial shunt infection, the isolation of the offending organism from the blood may be made more likely by pumping the shunt flushing chamber several times immediately before drawing blood.

Staphylococci from the blood of a patient with a shunt colonization may appear to be mixed on first isolation, and this is especially so in long-standing ventriculo–atrial shunt infections or after antibiotic treatment. This is due to variations in colony size and a mixture of three or four strains may be suggested. However, when the different colonies are subcultured, they often give rise to the same mixture of colony sizes, or they may well revert to a more usual appearance suggesting a pure culture. The appearance on first isolation should therefore never be taken as evidence of a mixed culture and, by implication, contamination. Biotyping usually indicates a pure culture in genuine shunt colonization, though mixed infections with two species of coagulase-negative staphylococci occasionally occur.

Cerebrospinal fluid aspiration

Aspiration of cerebrospinal fluid from the shunt system for diagnostic purposes is a relatively simple manoeuvre, but because of the risk of introducing bacteria it should only be carried out when shunt colonization is suspected on other grounds, and then using strict aseptic technique. Coagulase-negative staphylococci and coryneforms are usually present in large numbers on healthy scalp (Marples, 1965; Noble, 1981) and there is no way of eradicating them completely prior to skin puncture. Their numbers may be decreased by thorough preparation on the site using alcoholic povidone-iodine, preferably preceded by a small povidone-iodine dressing for a few hours. However, due to the risk of contaminating the aspirate with povidone-iodine, thorough cleansing with an isopropyl alcohol swab may be preferred.

Myers and Schoenbaum (1975) performed aspiration of the valve chamber or reservoir in 64 patients suspected of having colonized shunts, and cultures were made on 59 of these. The causative organism was isolated in 24 of 25 patients not receiving antibiotics, and in 18 of 34 patients to whom antibiotics were being administered. Cases of proven shunt colonization have also been encountered where shunt aspiration was negative while the patients were receiving antibiotics for suspected intercurrent infections. As shunt aspiration is often regarded as a definitive procedure, this may lead to wrong diagnosis if the suppressive effect of the antibiotics is not appreciated and taken into account.

The site of the puncture depends to a large extent on the type of shunting device used. If there is a flushing chamber such as is found in Ames or Holter shunts, this may be used for aspiration. If there is a reservoir in addition to a flushing chamber, such as in a Holter shunt fitted with a Rickham reservoir or a Hakim shunt, then the latter is usually chosen, but there is no reason why the Holter flushing chamber should not be tapped. If reasonable care is taken it is very difficult to damage the valves and the chamber does not leak after tapping any more readily than a reservoir, provided a fine needle, preferably of the Huber type, is used.

In shunt systems employing proximal valves and where the reservoir is proximally placed in relation to these, as in the Rickham–Holter system above, then a misleading result may arise from tapping either the reservoir or the flushing chamber. In a recent study, 10 shunts, removed because of colonization, were examined to determine the site of the colonization (Bayston and Spitz, 1978). None of the patients had ventriculitis. In 5 of 6 ventriculo–atrial shunts the valves, flushing chamber and lower catheter were colonized, but not the ventricular catheter. In the sixth case, only the catheter distal to the slit valves was colonized. In this patient the colonization arose when the distal catheter was electively lengthened. Had the diagnosis depended on a tap of either the reservoir or the flushing chamber, the negative results obtained might have allowed the distal catheter colonization to go undetected. In the remaining 4 ventriculoperitoneal shunts, 3 had colonization confined to the distal catheter. This is usual where the primary procedure is a ventriculo–atrial shunt and revision, usually involving only the distal catheter, is to a ventriculoperitoneal shunt. Again, the diagnosis would have been missed if it had depended on aspiration of the reservoir or the flushing chamber. Retrograde migration of staphylococci up Holter shunts appears to be reliably prevented by the slit valves, as shown by both laboratory and clinical studies (Bayston and Spitz, 1978). Indeed, in 1 case of ventriculoperitoneal shunt referred to above where colonization was found to involve the ventricular catheter and flushing chamber as well as the distal catheter, the slit valves were both found to allow reflux on testing.

When fluid which has been aspirated from a shunt is examined in the laboratory, both aerobic and anaerobic culture should be set up (Everett, Eickhoff and Simon, 1976; Brook *et al.*, 1980), and a total and differential cell count should be done. A Gram-stained film should always be examined for organisms, as this often allows an early diagnosis to be made without awaiting culture results. It is also invaluable in differentiating contamination from infection. The former is usually due to a small number of organisms, usually too few to be detected on Gram film, whereas true colonization involves a much greater number of organisms which in our experience can almost always be seen in Gram film. Expressed differently, a positive culture report in the presence of a negative Gram film is extremely suggestive of contamination.

As previously stated, in cases of suspected shunt colonization, examination of aspirated cerebrospinal fluid may be negative where the patient is receiving antibiotics, perhaps for an intercurrent infection. In such cases, repeat aspiration should be performed a few days after cessation of treatment. Myers and Schoenbaum (1975) found all of 4 Gram films on fluid taken from patients not on antibiotics to be positive, but only 2 of 4 patients who were taking antibiotics and who had proven shunt infection. It is noteworthy that a third patient in this group had a diagnostically positive Gram film in the presence of negative cultures of aspirate and blood.

If there is pleocytosis, and Gram films and cultures fail to show evidence of infection, other causes for this should be considered. Metrizamide is known to give rise to cerebrospinal fluid pleocytosis, and raised intracranial pressure and intracranial ischaemia or hypoxia may lead to demyelination which in turn may lead to cerebrospinal fluid pleocytosis. If a film is dried, fixed in formalin and stained for lipid using Scarlet R, a high proportion of the cells may be found to contain myelin-derived fat (Chester, Penny and Emery, 1971). Where *Staphylococcus aureus* shunt infection is suspected, this is often confined to the external surfaces of the shunt and shunt aspiration may be contraindicated due to the risk of disseminating sepsis into the central nervous system.

Examination of removed shunts

All cerebrospinal fluid shunts and catheters removed at operation should be examined bacteriologically. If this is done correctly as described below, not only is a valuable definitive diagnosis available but colonization is detected in some cases where it was previously unsuspected. The underlying pathology which made shunting necessary often makes clinical diagnosis of shunt infection difficult, especially as the classic features are frequently absent in the early stages. Malfunctioning ventriculo–atrial shunts are frequently revised to ventriculoperitoneal, and malfunctioning ventriculo-peritoneal shunts are often resited in the abdomen after freeing of adhesions. In the absence of serological studies (Bayston, 1975; Bayston and Spitz, 1977; Bayston and Swinden, 1979) shunt infection may not be suspected prior to surgical removal or revision for malfunction. However, an infected ventriculoperitoneal shunt which is merely resited will usually require re-operation in a matter of weeks because of peritonitis or malfunction due to peritoneal cyst formation (Bayston and Spitz, 1977).

Partial revision of an infected ventriculo–atrial shunt for malfunction will lead to persistence of the infection and, if this continues to go unrecognized, to immune complex nephritis (Black, Challacombe and Ockenden, 1965; Bayston and Swinden, 1979). The need for bacteriological examination of removed shunts is therefore evident. However, unnecessary extension of hospital stay and antibiotic therapy and in some cases unnecessary surgery, may be a consequence of cultural methods which yield results suggesting infection which are in fact due to contamination. For these reasons above, it is considered that careful examination of all removed shunt components, irrespective of the reasons for removal, is essential.

Another reason is the need for collection of accurate data on shunt infections, particularly where these form a part of the national statistics. It is believed that, due to the lack of reliable clinical information or lack of time to obtain it, many such statistics are based solely on the results of the conventional method of examination, which may not be capable of differentiating contamination from infection.

In many laboratories removed shunts are merely immersed in broth and subcultured after incubation (Bayston *et al.*, 1983). The culture media and incubation time vary and anaerobic cultures are usually omitted. Surgical incisions have been shown to become contaminated with skin flora during operation (Ives and Hirshfeld, 1939; Velghe, Dereymaeker and van der Voorde, 1964; Raahave, 1976) and this has been found to occur in shunt operations in at least 60% of cases (Bayston and Lari, 1974). It is therefore not unreasonable to expect the external surfaces of shunts to be contaminated to some extent during removal. The isolation of skin bacteria from shunts which have been incubated in broth as described above, is therefore considered to be at best meaningless and at worst misleading.

The method of examination used in this laboratory is designed to produce results relating to shunt colonization rather than to chance contamination. The shunt should be removed with minimum of manipulation and immediately placed intact into a sterile jar which is large enough to accept it without cramming. It should then either be sent to the laboratory or refrigerated at +4°C until this is possible.

In the laboratory, the shunt should be transferred using sterile forceps to a sterile stainless-steel dish and examined. After a brief description has been noted, any purulent material on the external surface is swabbed for microscopy and culture. An area on the external surface of each shunt component is then thoroughly cleaned using a swab soaked in isopropyl alcohol, and fluid is aspirated from the lumen using a sterile syringe and needle. If no fluid is obtainable the component may be irrigated with a small volume of sterile saline solution. Culture broths should not be used for irrigation since they often contain dead bacteria originating from the dehydrated powder

TABLE 3.3
Results of bacteriological examination of 55 shunts

Method	Total positive	Clinically infected
A	9	8
B	31	7
A alone	1	1
B alone	23	0

TABLE 3.4
Results of positives by Method A, all clinically infected

Patient	Site	Gram	Culture
BD*	LC	+C+++	NG
KD	VC, V	+C++++	*Staph. aureus*
EC	VC	+C++++	Coagulase-negative staphylococci
LS	VC	+C+, −B+	*Staph. aureus, Ps. aeruginosa*
	V	+C+	*Staph. aureus*
EP* (2)°	VC	+C+	NG
PC	VC, V, LC	+C++	Coagulase-negative staphylococci
RM (2)°	VC, LC	+C++	Coagulase-negative staphylococci
NC*	VC	NOS	Coagulase-negative staphylococci

VC ventricular catheter; LC lower catheter; V valve chamber; NG no growth.
+C Gram-positive cocci; −B Gram-negative bacilli; NOS no organisms seen.
* Patient on antibiotics.,
° The second of two revisions.

or granules from which they are reconstituted, and these can be grossly misleading on microscopy. The fluid obtained from each component is used to make a Gram film and to inoculate a cooked meat or thioglycollate medium, and a blood agar plate. A sterile Pasteur pipette may be used instead of a syringe and needle if only open-ended catheters are submitted for examination, but care must be taken not to contaminate the aspirate from the external surface of the catheter.

The author has recently conducted a comparison of this method (Method A) with the conventional broth culture procedure (Method B) (Bayston *et al.*, 1983). The results of bacteriological examination of 55 CSF shunts are shown in Tables 3.3 and 3.4. Nine shunts were considered positive by Method A and 8 of these were clinically infected. The exception (RM) had two revisions. At the first revision coagulase-negative staphylococcus was isolated by Method A but only on secondary culture. The Gram film was negative and there was no clinical evidence of shunt infection. Patient NC was also negative by Gram film but positive on culture by Method A. Patient BD and Patient EP (second revision) had organisms in the Gram film but culture by Method A was negative, probably because they were receiving antibiotics.

Eight of the 9 shunts which were positive by Method A were positive by Method B; the exception was patient BD. The most important finding was that 23 shunts were positive by Method B only, and none of these was clinically infected.

Table 3.4 shows the detailed results of examination of the 8 infected shunts by Method A. One was due to *Staphylococcus aureus*, 4 were due to coagulase-negative staphylococci and in 2 no organisms were isolated though they were seen in the Gram film. One patient (LS) had a grossly infected extracranial collection of cerebrospinal fluid around the shunt which yielded 5 organisms when aspirated preoperatively. *Staphylococcus aureus* was isolated from the fluid from the valve chamber, and *Staphylococcus aureus* and *Pseudomonas aeruginosa* were isolated from the fluid in the upper catheter. The shunt was shown to be malfunctioning.

Table 3.5 shows the detailed results of those shunts which were positive by Method B, and culture results by Method A are included for comparison. Patient BD, who was clincially infected and whose shunt fluid microscopy was positive but whose culture by both methods failed to grow any organism, is included for completeness. On the basis of sensitypes, it can be seen that the same strain which was isolated in the infected cases by Method A was also isolated by Method B, though the latter method often yielded more than one organism. The results show that the conventional method of examining removed shunts yielded positive cultures from 42% whereas the use of Method A resulted in 16% which showed organisms either by microscopy or on culture of the fluid inside the shunt. In 3 patients with shunt infections who were receiving antibiotics there was no correlation between microscopy and culture by Method A. In one case (BD) the infection would not have been detected had microscopy been omitted.

In a further case RM (first revision), examination using Method A showed no organisms in the Gram film or on the primary culture but grew coagulase-negative staphylococcus (sensitype 440) from the secondary culture only. This strain, along with another was isolated

Diagnosis of shunt infection

TABLE 3.5
Comparison of the culture results of CSF shunts by two methods

Patient	Site	Culture (Method B)	Culture (Method A)
HD	LC	Coag.-neg.staph. 200	NG
CO	VC, LC	Coag.-neg.staph. 400	NG
CB	VC	Coag.-neg.staph. 410, Diphtheroid	NG
JP	LC	Coag.-neg.staph. 402	NG
KD	VC	Coag.-neg.staph. 400	NG
UC	VC	Coag.-neg.staph. 410, 500, 600	NG
KD*	VC, V	*Staph. aureus* 400	*Staph. aureus* 400
CO	VC, V, LC	*Staph. aureus* 610, *Bacillus sp.*	NG
EC*	VC	Coag.-neg.staph. 443, 662	Coag.-neg.staph. 443
JG	LC	Coag.-neg.staph. 600	NG
SP	VC, V	Coag.-neg.staph. 440, 540	NG
CO	VC	Diphtheroid	NG
FA	VC	*Micrococcus sp.* 000	NG
DT	V, LC	Coag.-neg.staph. 000	NG
DB	VC, V	Coag.-neg.staph. 400	NG
EP (1)	LC	Coag.-neg.staph. 400	NG
LS*	VC, V	*Staph. aureus* 410	*Staph. aureus* 410
		Ps. aeruginosa	*Ps. aeruginosa*
		Klebsiella, E. coli, Strep. faecalis	
EP (2)*	UC	Coag.-neg.staph. 453	NG (Gram film +C +)
PC*	VC, V, LC	Coag.-neg.staph. 000	Coag.-neg.staph. 000
SA	V, LC	Coag.-neg.staph. 000	NG
MG	VC	Coag.-neg.staph. 400	NG
RM (1)	VC, V	Coag.-neg.staph. 400, 440	2° Culture only coag.-neg.staph. 440
CS	VC, V, LC	Coag.-neg.staph. 400, Diphtheroid	NG
DM	LC	Coag.-neg.staph. 020	NG
NB	LC	Coag.-neg.staph. 000.010.420, 600	NG
RM (2)*	VC, LC	Coag.-neg.staph. 000,440	
		Strep. viridans	NG
JB	VC	Coag.-neg.staph. 000	NG
DM	LC	Coag.-neg.staph. 510, 650	
		Bacillus sp. ×2	NG
SA	VC	Coag.-neg.staph. 020	NG
DP	VC	Coag.-neg.staph. 000	NG
NC*	VC	Coag.-neg.staph. 510	Coag.-neg.staph. 510
BD*	LC	NG	NG (Gram film +C +++)

Coag.-neg.staph. Coagulase-negative staphylococci.
* Clinically infected cases.
Numbers following organisms refer to sensitype.
Other abbreviations as in Table 3.4.

by Method B. The patient later developed features of shunt colonization and coagulase-negative staphylococcus, sensitype 440, was
isolated from the ventricular fluid before shunt removal as well as

from the fluid inside the second removed shunt (Table 3.5). While it is impossible to say whether the first shunt from which growth was obtained only on subculture was infected, it is considered more likely that the fluid inside the removed shunt was accidentally contaminated either by organisms in the incision, or by organisms from the outer surface of the shunt. The subsequent infection of the second shunt was probably due to its contamination during revision, also by organisms present in the incision, and it would not therefore be surprising that the same organisms were involved in these events.

None of those cases positive only by Method B showed evidence of infection. Presumably at least some of those which yielded pure cultures using Method B would have been reported as shunt infection by laboratories using this method.

The examination of a Gram film is important, and this view is supported by the two cases where organisms were seen on microscopy but failed to grow on culture due to antibiotic treatment. Another reason for the inclusion of the Gram film is that some organisms responsible for shunt infections may require more than two days' incubation to grow, and this is particularly true of some coryneforms (Everett, Eickhoff and Simon, 1976). Where such organisms are seen in a Gram film of intraluminal fluid, culture methods may be changed or incubation times extended in order to ensure their isolation. For example *Propionibacterium acnes* is an occasional but important cause of shunt infection and prolonged anaerobic culture has been recommended (Beeler *et al.*, 1976) where the presence of this organism is suspected.

Shunt infections may be divided into two groups. The first group, external to the shunt and not extending to its lumen, are usually caused by *Staphylococcus aureus* or coliforms. These are really wound infections or rarely secondarily infected collections of cerebrospinal fluid. In such cases the fluid inside the shunt will give negative results unless either the shunt lumen has become infected before removal by needle aspiration through the infected area, or has been contaminated in the laboratory by organisms from the external surfaces of the shunt. As such external infections are almost always clinically obvious, and pus can usually be aspirated or collected at operation, the exclusive use of Method A should still result in their being detected and properly investigated.

External infection should be suspected clinically preoperatively and determined at operation, when swabs can be taken for culture.

The second group, designated internal infections, which are far more common in most units and are usually due to coagulase-negative staphylococci, coryneforms or propionibacteria, represent true shunt infection. The author's results suggest that, in this group, the exclusive use of Method B will result in overdiagnosis of shunt infection, whereas the use•of both methods, or preferably the exclusive use of Method A will yield more accurate information on which to base a diagnosis. In a study conducted by Fokes (1970), shunt components removed at operation were placed in culture broth and subcultured after incubation. In 6 patients who had no clinical or laboratory evidence of shunt infection before revision, some part of the removed shunt grew either coagulase-negative staphylococci or coryneforms, and Fokes describes this as 'a third clinically inapparent form of ventriculo–atrial shunt infection', the first and second being early and late infections. With the possible exception of one case the most likely explanation of Fokes' findings is that he had isolated organisms which had contaminated the outer surface of the shunt tubing during removal, or possibly which had contaminated the tubing or culture broth in the laboratory.

As with blood cultures from shunted patients, unusual or 'commensal' organisms should not be disregarded as contaminants unless there is good evidence for this. Careful technique involving luminal fluid culture should reduce contamination to a minimum and the routine use of the direct gram film will allow correct interpretation of those few cases which do occur.

Serum antibody tests – rationale and development

It has been seen that clinical manifestations of shunt colonization are very variable and can be misleading, and that blood culture is not a reliable diagnostic tool even in ventriculo–atrial shunts. Morrice and Young (1974) state that, in one of their studies, actual diagnosis of shunt colonization was not easy until the shunt was removed and cultured. Where evidence such as a single positive blood culture has been accepted as diagnostic of shunt colonization, the shunt has sometimes, in our experience, shown no sign of colonization when examined in the laboratory after removal. A competent shunt should be preserved if possible, and more reliable evidence of the presence of colonization should be required before the decision to remove it is made.

The use of a test for circulating antibody as a diagnostic tool was first considered in relation to the difficulty of distinguishing 'contaminants' from 'pathogens' in blood cultures (Bayston, 1971); that is, if an organism isolated from a blood culture was present as a pathogen, the patient should react to its presence by producing antibody whereas, of course, if the isolate were a contaminant this would not be so. Using a strain of coagulase-negative staphylococcus of Baird–Parker–Holt type SIIA, a type commonly found in colonized shunts (Holt, 1969), and a serum sample from a patient known to have a colonized ventriculo–atrial shunt due to coagulase-negative staphylococcus, tests for antibody–antigen interaction were carried out with little initial success.

The reaction between staphylococci isolated from patients with septicaemia and homologous serum was tested by Smith *et al.* (1958), and the results were discouraging in that very low titres were found. This relative lack of antigenicity which was also found in the author's experiments (Bayston, 1972), was originally thought to be to a non-antigenic surface component which blocked the reaction. This blocking substance was thought to be mucopeptide in nature, and was thought to be analogous to the mucoid surface substance (slime) described in connection with adherence of the organisms to the luminal surface of shunts (Bayston and Penny, 1972).

Various ways of removing this substance were investigated, and the simplest and most effective was prolonged heating. After such treatment, the agglutinability of the strains improved markedly and high titres of antibody could be demonstrated in some sera. Moreover, the exposed surface antigen was found to be common to virtually all strains of coagulase-negative staphylococci. Only two strains of SVI, a type which we rarely isolated, were unreactive. *Staphylococcus aureus* and most strains of micrococcus did not react with sera raised against this SIIA antigen in rabbits, though a few have since been found to cross-react. When sera of 509 children were tested using this antigen, high titres were found in 9 children, all of whom had proven shunt colonization due to coagulase-negative staphylococcus (Bayston, 1972).

Method of test for antibody in coagulase-negative staphylococcus

The method of production of antigen is very simple. A stock laboratory strain of SIIA, which was originally isolated from a colonized shunt, is inoculated onto several horse blood agar plates and incubated at 37°C for 48 hours. The incubation period is important as the antigens utilized in the test are expressed only after this duration. The growth is then washed off with phosphate buffered saline (PBS), pH 7.3, with the aid of a bent glass rod and washed by centrifuging twice in PBS. The deposit is then re-suspended in about 5 ml of PBS and autoclaved at 121°C for 1 hour. Significant deviation from this temperature and time lead to lower agglutinability. The suspension is then washed again in PBS and the deposit re-suspended in about 5 ml PBS as a stock concentrate and kept at +4°C. For use, a quantity of the concentrate is diluted in 20 ml of PBS to give a suspension of 80% absorbance at wavelength 601 nm.

It is important to use PBS of pH 7.3. Physiological saline solution for clinical use has a lower pH which causes difficulty in reading end-points.

The titration is best carried out in plastic microtitre trays (e.g. Cooke) with rows of twelve U-shaped wells. Using an automatic pipette (e.g. Finnpipette), 100 μl of PBS are dispensed into each well, and a further 100 μl into the first well. Twenty microlitres of test serum are then added to the first well. Using the 100 μl automatic pipette, this is mixed and 100 μl transferred to the second well, and so on using doubling dilutions and discarding 100 μl from the twelfth well after mixing. Each well now contains 100 μl and the reciprocal dilutions of serum range from 10 to 20 480. One hundred microlitres of diluted antigen are then added to each well, making the final dilutions range from 20 to 40 960. Control sera having titres of, for example, 80 and 2560, are put up with each test batch. The microtitre tray is covered and refrigerated at +4°C overnight, after which the results are readable following a period of a few minutes at 37°C at room temperature to allow condensation to be removed from the underside of the tray. Reading is facilitated by using a specially designed reader such as the 'Titertek' (Flow Laboratories)*. The highest dilution giving 100% agglutination, with no trace of a 'button' is taken as the end-point.

Interpretation

It is important to realize that, except for very young children, the serum will contain some antibody to coagulase-negative staphylococci and the titre has been shown to rise with age until about the

---

* Flow Laboratories Ltd, PO Box 17, Second Avenue, Industrial Estate, Irvine, Ayrshire, Scotland KA12 8NB.

third or fourth year (Bayston, 1975; Holt, 1980). Sera from 297 children, aged from 2 weeks to 15 years, 100 of whom did not have hydrocephalus and all of whom were considered to be free of shunt colonization, were tested. In children of less than 6 months of age in both groups the titres were usually 20 or less. The titres then rose steadily with age in both groups, and the mean titre levelled off in both groups at a mean of 160 after between 3 and 4 years. Titres of up to 640 may be found in adults and up to 1280 in the elderly.

These cross-sectional data have been confirmed many times by longitudinal studies. This is helpful in interpretation of single titres, as a 6-month-old child with a titre of 160, a 5-year-old child with a titre of 640, and a 25-year-old adult with a titre of 2560, may all be said to show abnormally high antibody levels. However, interpretation is made much easier in the individual case by having a baseline result so that a rise in titre may be detected. This may be accomplished by habitually estimating the titre as part of the preoperative work-up, and is even more effective if a surveillance scheme is employed (see Chapter 4).

The serum antibody titre rarely rises significantly in patients with colonized ventriculoperitoneal shunts, and it also sometimes fails to rise in ventriculitis due to coagulase-negative staphylococci, even in the presence of a ventriculo–atrial shunt. The reasons for this are not currently understood, but the finding is consistent, and is probably partly due to the early presentation in most cases.

However, in both these cases, the serum C-reactive protein test is positive unless the patient is receiving antibiotics. Titres in patients with longstanding ventriculo–atrial shunt colonization commonly range from 1280 to > 40 960. Though neonates do not naturally have detectable antibody (it would appear that maternal antibody is not transmitted in this case) they, along with infants, are capable of mounting a vigorous antibody response to a colonized ventriculo–atrial shunt. Titres can be depressed temporarily by the use of oral cloxacillin or by other antibiotic regimens which suppress the bacteraemia, and the occasional patient with a colonized, blocked shunt who is not shunt-dependent and is usually asymptomatic may consistently show a normal titre. In such cases, the titre often rises rapidly to abnormal levels after shunt revision, presumably due to release of antigen from the shunt into the bloodstream during operation.

It is also noteworthy that, in those patients whose titres have remained at very high levels after eradication of the colonization, the titres may remain high for two years or more. This is probably due to fixation of antigen in the tissues and should not be taken as indicative of persisting colonization, which usually results in a further rise in titre. Patients' sera may be tested for antibody to other bacteria in the same way as that described, but where this has been attempted the strain of organism isolated from the patient has to be used as it has been found that organisms such as *Escherichia coli* and *Staphylococcus aureus* do not possess antigens common to most strains in their genera. However, while serological tests may not be very useful diagnostically in such cases, titres may fall rapidly during treatment and they have been found useful for monitoring purposes and for early detection of relapse.

C-reactive protein test

C-reactive protein (CRP) is so called because it was originally thought to be found only in patients with pneumococcal pneumonia. The protein, present in the 'acute phase' serum of these patients, reacted strongly with the pneumococcal capsular polysaccharide, hence the term 'C (for capsular)-reactive' (Tillet and Francis, 1930). Originally it was thought to be absent from the serum of healthy individuals, but more sensitive tests have shown that it is always present, though the levels are much lower in health. Measurements of serum CRP have been used to assess the severity of the disease process and to monitor treatment in rheumatic fever (Anderson and McCarty, 1950), and other workers have used it in other inflammatory conditions (Bunim *et al.*, 1952).

CRP is one of a group of acute-phase reactants. The concentration of these substances in the plasma rises or falls in response to cell damage. Examples are α_1-antitrypsin and α_2-macroglobulin, which prevent further cell damage by binding lysosomal enzymes. The plasma concentration of CRP rises after cell damage, and while its precise function is not known for certain it may be assumed to have some beneficial role in either prevention of secondary damage or in repair.

There is also evidence that it may enhance the lytic functions of the complement system. After cell damage has taken place, for example due to accidental trauma or sepsis, the parenchymal cells in the liver begin to produce increased amounts of the acute-phase reactants. The plasma concentrations change at different rates (Figure 3.1) and

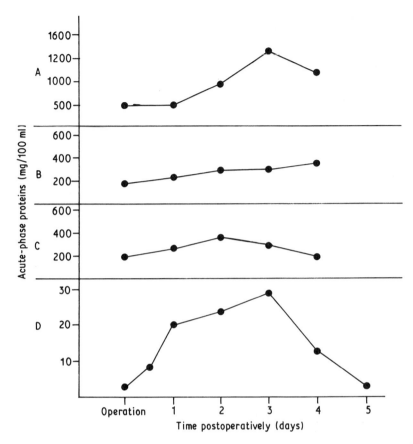

Figure 3.1 Reactions of some acute-phase proteins to operation. A α_1-acid glycoprotein; B haptoglobin; C α_1-antitrypsin; D C-reactive protein.

the concentration of CRP is the first to rise (Rapport, Schwartz and Graf, 1957; Crockson *et al.*, 1966; Fischer *et al.*, 1976; Bayston, 1979).

The serum CRP level has been observed to rise following surgery, and has been used for monitoring postoperative progress and for early detection of postoperative complications (Fischer *et al.*, 1976). The author has used this test alongside the coagulase-negative staphylococcus antibody test in the diagnosis of cerebrospinal fluid shunt infections. The results to be expected in patients undergoing shunt surgery and whose postoperative course is uneventful are shown in Figure 3.2. The CRP level rises after ventriculo–atrial shunt insertions, and falls to normal in two or three days, whereas it usually rises higher after ventriculoperitoneal shunt insertion and after

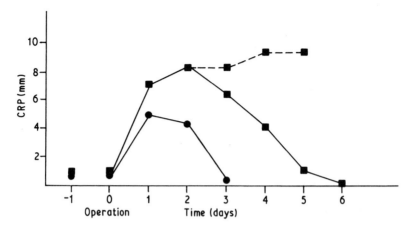

Figure 3.2 CRP results following shunt surgery. ● ● VA shunt insertion;
■ ■ VP shunt insertion; ■ ■ colonized VP shunt. CRP measured in mm
by capillary precipitation method.

revision of a ventriculo–atrial shunt to a ventriculoperitoneal shunt,
and takes longer to fall to normal. The amount of tissue damage is
greater in ventriculoperitoneal shunt insertions due to the subcutaneous tunnelling entailed in placement of the distal catheter, and
this almost certainly accounts for the slightly prolonged high CRP
levels in patients undergoing this operation.

Having established the normal pattern, one can use CRP tests to
detect complications of shunt surgery (Bayston, 1979; Castro-Gago
et al., 1982). The results in a series of 120 patients admitted to
hospital with suspected shunt sepsis are shown in Table 3.6. None of
those subsequently found to have ventriculo–atrial shunt infection
due to coagulase-negative staphylococci without ventriculitis or
shunt nephritis had a positive CRP test, whereas all those with
ventriculoperitoneal shunt infection due to these organisms gave a
positive test. In early uncomplicated ventriculo–atrial shunt infection due to coagulase-negative staphylococci, the inflammatory
response is slight, the symptoms are often mild and there is rarely
evidence of metastatic sepsis. The normal CRP levels are consistent
to these observations. In ventriculoperitoneal shunt infections due to
coagulase-negative staphylococci, there is an inflammatory reaction
in the peritoneal cavity and often erythema over the track of the distal
catheter. Again, the CRP would be expected to be positive in this
condition.

TABLE 3.6
C-reactive protein results in patients with suspected shunt sepsis

Final diagnosis	Number of patients	Positive (%)	Negative
Uncomplicated, 'early' VA Shunt infection (coagulase-negative staphylococci)	36	0	36
Shunt nephritis	19	19 (100)	0
Ventriculitis (coagulase-negative staphylococci)	11	8 (73)	3
VP shunt infection (coagulase-negative staphylococci)	40	40 (100)	0
VP or VA shunt infection (*Staph. aureus*)	8	8 (100)	0
V-PL shunt infection (coagulase-negative staphylococci)	3	3 (100)	0
Urinary tract infection*	11	7 (64)	4
Respiratory tract infection*	12	9 (75)	3
Otitis media*	6	5 (83)	1
Totals	146	99	47

VA ventriculo–atrial; VP ventriculoperitoneal; VPL ventriculopleural.
* These were severe, with general toxicity.

Staphylococcus aureus infection of both types of shunt system normally gives rise to a vigorous inflammatory response with cellular necrosis mediated by the toxins produced by the organism, and the CRP is consistently highly positive in such cases. This is also true of infections due to organisms such as pseudomonas and the proteus group.

Shunt nephritis represents a chronic inflammatory lesion, and the serum CRP level is always moderately raised while this lesion remains active.

Of the 29 patients who were found to have infections of the respiratory or urinary tracts or the middle ear, 21 gave a positive serum CRP test. In bacterial respiratory tract infections, serum CRP levels are known to rise rapidly, and this has been suggested as a means of differentiating them from infections of viral origin (Kindmark, 1976). Similarly, in children with urinary tract infection a raised CRP is said to be a good indicator of renal involvement.

The CRP test is certainly not specific, but when carried out alongside the coagulase-negative staphylococcus antibody test as part of the usual battery of investigations carried out on a shunted patient with fever, it proves invaluable. Cystic malfunction of infective origin in ventriculoperitoneal shunts is easily distinguished from that which is not associated with sepsis (Figure 3.2) whereas this diagnosis might otherwise be missed, leading to repeated recurrence (Bayston and Spitz, 1977). Shunt sepsis should be strongly suspected in a patient with ventriculoperitoneal shunt, who, within two or three months of shunt surgery and not having taken antibiotics, presents with fever, abdominal pain or discomfort and signs of shunt malfunction, and has a positive serum CRP test. Other possible causes for the raised CRP level such as infections of the urinary or respiratory tracts are capable of easy and rapid exclusion by routine tests and clinical examination.

Similarly, a patient with a ventriculo–atrial shunt which has been in position for one to two years or more, who presents with fever and has a high coagulase-negative staphylococcus antibody titre, and in addition a positive CRP test, will often be found to have not only a colonized shunt but at least urinary if not clinical evidence of shunt nephritis. Such serological information may be the first indication of immune complex nephritis in a patient whose longstanding shunt colonization has not previously been diagnosed because of unconvincing symptoms and omission of serological tests.

CRP may be detectable in cerebrospinal fluid, particularly in cases of bacterial meningitis (Corrall *et al.*, 1981) but CRP is not thought to be synthesized within the central nervous system and its presence in cerebrospinal fluid must be considered to be due to the increased vascular permeability in bacterial meningitis.

If the cerebrospinal fluid CRP test is incorporated into a CIE (countercurrent immunoelectrophoresis) system such as that commonly used to detect bacterial antigens, or similar latex agglutination tests, then positive cerebrospinal fluid results may be obtained in cases of bacterial meningitis when the patient's serum is negative for CRP using a different test system. This may be due to difference in test sensitivity, but it may also be due to slower elimination of CRP from the cerebrospinal fluid than from serum.

A variety of techniques are available for measurement of serum CRP. Quantitative methods include immunoelectrophoresis and radial immunodiffusion. Both methods are simple, precise and sensitive, but immunoelectrophoresis is more rapid. However, the author has found a semiquantitative capillary precipitation method to be satisfactory. No equipment is required and all the reagents and capillary tubes are supplied in kit form. The test requires approximately 25 µl of serum and the relatively low sensitivity of the test means that most sera containing normal CRP concentrations appear negative. Results are normally read after reacting overnight, but these may be read after three to five hours at 37°C. Serum must be used as CRP binds to heparin and other anticoagulants are said to interfere. The test is carried out using antiserum to CRP (Difco Laboratories*). Capillary tubes, supplied with the kit, are marked at 4 cm and 8 cm with a spirit pen, leaving 1 cm at one end, and 25 µl of anti-CRP antiserum is run up to the 4 cm mark, followed by an equal volume of patient's serum. The tube is then rocked several times using the remaining 1 cm to mix the two sera, and plunged into a block of modelling clay (Plasticine) so that the foot of the fluid column is still visible. The tube is left at room temperature overnight.

When CRP is present in detectable quantities in the patient's serum it combines with the antibody in the antiserum to form a precipitate which falls to the foot of the column. The height of the precipitate is measured in millimetres and the result may be expressed as such, but it is more usually expressed as the number of millimetres followed by a 'plus' sign: 2 mm=2+, 5 mm=5+. Sera giving results of 2+ contain about 12 mg/dl of CRP, and those giving 5+ contain about 130 mg/dl.

The CRP test has for some reason become an emotive issue with many deciding against it on the grounds that it is non-specific. These unscientific assessments are fuelled by reports of its irrelevance from those who do not take into account the timing of the samples and the fact that, though it is certainly a non-specific indicator of tissue damage, intelligent assessment of the meaning of results in individual patients can be very useful. If a patient with a ventriculoperitoneal shunt in place for less than six months has a positive CRP test and no obvious cause can be found on clinical examination and simple laboratory tests, then shunt infection should be suspected. Further action should include repeat of the test on a second sample and careful observation of the patient at more frequent clinic visits over the following few weeks. If the second sample is positive or if clinical evidence is found then shunt colonization should be assumed until excluded. A negative result in a suspected case is also very helpful.

* Difco Laboratories, PO Box 14B, Central Avenue, East Molesey, Surrey, KT8 0SE.

Serum complement levels in shunt nephritis

The original report of shunt nephritis (Black, Challacombe and Ockenden, 1965) described the deposition of immunoglobulins and complement on the basement membranes of the renal glomeruli, and this observation has since been confirmed several times.

After a prolonged period of immunization of the host due to release into the bloodstream of antigen from the colonized ventriculo–atrial shunt, the high antigen concentrations are matched by high antibody levels (Bayston and Swinden, 1979). The resulting circulating soluble immune complexes cause vasoactive peptides to be released from basophils and platelets. This causes separation of the endothelial cells, thus exposing the basement membranes. The larger complexes adhere to the exposed membranes and attract further deposits of immunoglobulins and complement. Neutrophils are attracted by chemotoxins and, in an attempt to phagocytose the fixed granules, release lysosomal enzymes which cause damage to the basement membranes resulting in microvascular thrombosis and haemorrhage, manifest clinically by glomerulonephritis. Some of the damage is also caused by the cytolytic activity of complement complexes.

Because of consumption of C_3, serum levels of this factor are depressed in shunt nephritis, and this is a useful diagnostic feature. It should be emphasized that, though congenital deficiences of complement components lead to increased susceptibility to infections, those with depressed serum levels which have been acquired due to, in this case, shunt nephritis are able to resist infections normally.

Various methods are available for the estimation of serum complement fractions. The method in common use for C_3 and C_4 fractions is based on that devised by Fahey and McKelvey (1965) for serum immunoglobulins. This consists of diffusion of serial dilutions of serum from wells cut in agar plates containing antibody to the substances sought. For C_3' and C_4', the appropriate reagents are substituted. The results are read in conjunction with controls and are usually expressed as a percentage of the 'normal' standard concentration.

3.5 SUMMARY

The clinical features of ventriculo–atrial shunt colonization differ from those of ventriculoperitoneal shunt colonization (Table 3.1). It is particularly important to note that early malfunction in ventriculo-peritoneal shunts is likely to have an infective cause. Shunt nephritis is caused by deposition of immune complexes and complement on the glomerular basement membranes. It is associated with delayed diagnosis of ventriculo–atrial shunt colonization and is therefore preventable. The diagnostic laboratory features are summarized in Table 3.2. When removed shunts or their components are examined in the laboratory for evidence of colonization, care should be taken to exclude contamination as this probably accounts for many of the unexpected 'positive' findings. Fluid should be aspirated aseptically for microscopical and cultural examination.

Any patient with a shunt who has a fever, and any patient with a ventriculoperitoneal shunt which repeatedly malfunctions or shows malfunction within two or three months of operation, should be suspected of having shunt colonization until this can be positively excluded.

4

SURVEILLANCE OF

PATIENTS AT RISK

The aetiology of shunt colonization has been discussed in Chapter 2. It has been seen that, at least those cases involving coagulase-negative staphylococci and probably also those involving coryneforms, are caused by organisms gaining access to the shunt during operation to insert or revise it. This timing of entry of the organisms is important when it comes to defining the period of risk of colonization to a patient with a cerebrospinal fluid shunt, and the implied time of risk is during the operation. Therefore, the presence of a shunt does not expose the patient to a continuing risk of colonization. It has also been seen that almost all so-called 'late' cases of shunt colonization have the same aetiology as 'early' ones but that for various reasons they are not detected promptly.

It has also been seen that the clinical features of shunt colonization are often present only intermittently and can be misleading, and that measurement of the serum coagulase-negative staphylococcus antibody titre and C-reactive protein level can be extremely useful in making an early diagnosis. This is preferable to waiting for months or years in patients with ventriculo–atrial shunts for the symptoms to become sufficiently convincing, by which time immunological complications may have begun to develop and the patient will have suffered an extended period of ill health, with deterioration of performance at school or at work, and accompanying strain on family and personal relationships. Unfortunately, such poor general health is expected by some patients and parents, and sadly by some clinicians, as an inevitable consequence of either shunting or the underlying condition.

While shunt serology is useful in resolving or confirming a diagnosis, it may be even more useful if carried out systematically and prospectively on all patients who undergo any kind of shunt surgery. In this way shunt colonization may be diagnosed serologically before the clinical features become obvious, and apart from the benefits outlined above, early diagnosis may be an important factor if non-surgical treatment is to be attempted (see Chapter 5). To this end a surveillance scheme, based on clinical interview and serological testing, has been designed (Bayston, 1975; Bayston and Swinden, 1979).

4.1   SURVEILLANCE SCHEME

The rationale and methodology of the coagulase-negative staphylo-coccus antibody and the serum C-reactive protein tests have been described in Chapter 3.

Timing of tests

For serological surveillance, these tests should be carried out pre-operatively for a baseline, and then approximately ten days post-operatively or before discharge from hospital, whichever is the sooner.

Thereafter, they are repeated at outpatient visits which should be arranged approximately one, three and six months after operation. At each visit, patients or their parents or guardians are interviewed about symptoms, based on those described in Chapter 3. In the author's experience it is logistically easier to carry out both antibody titre and C-reactive protein test on all patients regardless of which type of shunt system they have, but of course the interview should be structured to include questions particularly relevant to that patient's shunt system (see Chapter 3).

Other investigations such as blood culture, urine examination, blood count and fundoscopy may also be carried out at these sessions, at the clinician's discretion.

Results of tests

In a series of 488 children undergoing ventriculo–atrial shunt inser-tion or revision, many had preoperative and predischarge serology carried out, but only 127 had full surveillance for six months (Bayston and Swinden, 1979). The results in these two groups are

TABLE 4.1
Results of serological surveillance in children undergoing ventriculo–atrial
shunt surgery

	Surveillance	No surveillance
Number of cases	127	361
Number with 'early' colonization	7	3
Number with 'late' colonization	0	17
Number with shunt nephritis	1 (0.79%)	10 (3.6%)
Shunt colonization rate (%)	5.51	5.54

shown in Table 4.1. In the group which underwent surveillance, 7 patients were found to have colonized shunts, and all of these were diagnosed 'early', that is within the surveillance period.

One of these cases is discussed in Chapter 3. She remained very well but a rising antibody titre found on routine testing before discharge from hospital suggested shunt colonization with co-agulase-negative staphylococci. Blood cultures were intermittently positive, and she was slightly anaemic. However, she had already undergone multiple shunt revisions and further revision would have presented serious technical difficulties. Because of this, and because of her generally good condition, she was given oral cloxacillin and observed. Though her laboratory results showed gradually progress-ive abnormalities, she remained clinically well until she began to show signs of early shunt nephritis, with haematuria and depressed serum complement. Her antibody titre at this stage was more than 10 240 and her serum C-reactive protein level was abnormally high.

While this girl's shunt colonization was diagnosed early, technical surgical problems meant that no corrective action was possible and she was observed to pass from the stage of 'early' shunt colonization through 'late' shunt colonization at eighteen months after operation to shunt nephritis shortly afterwards. Had the surveillance results not been available, it is very likely that the diagnosis of this child's shunt colonization would not have been made until her health deteriorated enough to suggest investigation.

This case also illustrates that 'late' cases are in fact merely those 'early' ones where the diagnosis has not been made promptly, and that the availability of surveillance serology, even in those patients with no clinical evidence of shunt colonization, may mean that all cases are diagnosed 'early'. Indeed, in the group which did not undergo surveillance, of the 20 cases of shunt colonization 17 were 'late' diagnoses. Here the diagnosis was made on clinical grounds and serology was used only to confirm this. Of these 17, 10 children had evidence of shunt nephritis and 1 of these is known to have died of ensuing nephrotic syndrome.

The surveillance scheme is equally applicable to patients with ventriculoperitoneal shunts. In these cases the serum coagulase-negative staphylococcus antibody titre does not usually rise but the C-reactive protein level remains abnormally high or becomes so (see Chapter 3).

Also studied were 106 patients with ventriculoperitoneal shunts who underwent surveillance, and 41 subsequently developed distal end blockage (Bayston and Spitz, 1977). Ten of these 41 cases had high serum C-reactive protein levels within a few weeks of shunt surgery, and were subsequently found to have cystic blockage of infective origin. The remaining cases had negative C-reactive protein tests and presented between four months and seven years after surgery, with no evidence of sepsis.

One of the patients with cystic blockage of infective origin was mentioned in Chapter 3. She was asymptomatic but had a raised serum C-reactive protein level, and because of the lack of experience with serology at that time no immediate action was taken. Unfortunately, she became ill and died suddenly at home and necropsy confirmed infective cystic blockage of her ventriculoperitoneal shunt.

It may be seen from Chapter 3 that the serum C-reactive protein level rises in response to the trauma of shunt surgery, but this level should have returned to normal by the fifth postoperative day. If the shunt becomes colonized at the operation, the C-reactive protein level often remains elevated beyond the fifth postoperative day (see Figure 3.2), though it may return to normal temporarily only to rise again soon afterwards.

If prophylactic antimicrobials are used routinely to cover shunt surgery, this pattern of events may not apply, and the C-reactive protein level may return to normal, even in patients whose shunts are colonized, with a delayed rise later due to temporary suppression of infection by the antimicrobials.

One of the reasons for a surveillance system involving periodic investigations for six months following shunt surgery is that because of intervention such as antibacterial prophylaxis (or antimicrobial chemotherapy for an intercurrent infection, for example involving the urinary tract) or because of idiosyncrasy, or perhaps because of different virulence characteristics of the organisms involved, or variable shunt function (see Chapter 2), serological evidence of colonized shunt may appear either immediately after operation or at any time up to four or five months postoperatively.

Effects of surveillance

After applying the surveillance scheme to approximately 300 cases, three important conclusions have emerged. The first is that the application of the scheme allows reliable detection of shunt coloniz-ation in its early stages, often before definite symptoms appear, thus preventing the occurrence of secondary complications such as arth-ralgia and shunt nephritis. In ventriculoperitoneal shunts infection as a cause of malfunction can be clearly identified, thus modifying case management and avoiding repeated revisions. The second is that, if a patient reaches the end of the surveillance period without showing any clinical or serological evidence of shunt colonization, then he or she can be discharged from surveillance with confidence that the risk of shunt colonization has now passed and will not return until or unless further shunt surgery becomes necessary. This has been the author's constant finding, and a patient has not yet been seen who has passed successfully through the surveillance scheme who has developed 'late' shunt colonization.

Thirdly, the scheme must be administered by a competent person with sufficient experience and professional interest to monitor individual results closely, to build up and refer to a patient data base, and to discuss any and all anomalous results immediately with clinical colleagues. Only when administered in this way does a serological surveillance scheme, or even a serological diagnostic service, function satisfactorily.

Additionally, careful quality control of the tests is essential to detect and correct errors. While the tests are technically simple to perform, they should ideally be carried out by a reference centre for both the reasons stated above, and results should always be made available 24 hours after receipt of the sample.

4.2   SUMMARY

Diagnosis of shunt colonization can be made earlier and more accurately by the use of a serological surveillance scheme. This consists of a clinical interview and coagulase-negative staphylococcus antibody and serum C-reactive protein tests preoperatively, approximately ten days postoperatively or immediately before discharge from hospital, and then at outpatient visits at one, three and six months after operation. If there is no clinical or serological evidence of shunt colonization at this stage, the patient may be told that the likelihood of shunt colonization developing thereafter is so small that he need no longer worry about it. In practice, no patient has been seen who, having passed through the scheme, has later developed shunt colonization. 'Late' shunt colonization does not occur as a separate aetiological entity, and therefore complications such as shunt nephritis are not seen if diagnosis is made early.

4.3 RECOMMENDATIONS FOR CURRENT PRACTICE

1. Clotted blood, preferably 5 ml (minimum 0.5 ml) should be taken at the following intervals:
   (a) Preoperatively;
   (b) Ten days postoperatively or before discharge from hospital;
   (c) Four to six weeks postoperatively;
   (d) Three months postoperatively;
   (e) In patients with ventriculo–atrial shunts this should be extended to six months postoperatively.
2. Clinical interview and examination should be carried out at these intervals.
3. In patients with ventriculo–atrial shunts: if the antibody titre rises, even in the absence of symptoms, then blood culture and full blood count should be done and shunt tap should be considered. The patient should be examined thoroughly for signs of bacteraemia.
4. In patients with ventriculoperitoneal shunts: if the C-reactive protein level remains elevated beyond the sixth postoperative day, or if it rises again afterwards, then a non-shunt-related cause should be excluded. The patient should then be examined thoroughly for signs of shunt malfunction and of intra-abdominal inflammation. Shunt tap should be done but a negative result not taken to exclude shunt infection. Blood culture is unhelpful.

Extended observation, repeated clinical examination and repeat serology are recommended in doubtful cases.

5. If, at the end of the surveillance period, no serological or clinical evidence of shunt infection is found, then the likelihood of this developing is remote. This information can be transmitted to the patients or their parents or guardians in appropriate cases.

5

TREATMENT OF

SHUNT INFECTIONS

5.1 ALTERNATIVE TREATMENTS

The treatment of shunt infections may be surgical or non-surgical. In the surgical treatment, the shunt is removed, and this is followed by reshunting with or without intervening external ventricular drainage. In some cases further shunting will prove unnecessary. In the non-surgically treated cases, antibiotics are administered with the intention of eradicating the infection in the shunt and the tissues without recourse to shunt removal. Antibiotics are also used in conjunction with the surgical procedures, and most of the principles of antimicrobial chemotherapy which are particularly important in shunt infections apply equally to the surgical and the non-surgical approaches.

In cases which occurred soon after the first use of shunts for hydrocephalus, antibiotics were administered in the expectation that they would produce cure without surgery. This was based on lack of experience with shunt infections, and the view of coagulase-negative staphylococci as harmless commensal organisms of low virulence. Callaghan, Cohen and Stewart (1961) reported 5 children with ventriculo–atrial shunt infections, 3 due to coagulase-negative staphylococci and 2 due to *Staphylococcus aureus*. In 2 cases, methicillin was administered intravenously for long periods with no success, and the infected shunt eventually had to be removed. In another case, methicillin was not detectable in the cerebrospinal fluid during intravenous treatment, and this led to the decision to inject 3 mg of the drug daily into the ventricular system. On beginning intraventricular treatment the child's condition improved and he became apyrexial, but he later relapsed after treatment was stopped. Methicillin was used in the remaining 2 cases by both the intravenous and intraventricular routes with initial success followed by relapse requiring eventual removal of the shunt, even though intraventricular administration was continued for over 50 days. McLaurin (1973) reported 22 cases of shunt infection, 20 of which involved ventriculo–atrial shunts. Based on the premise that colonization occurs within the shunt tubing, and that therefore, antimicrobial drugs must reach the cerebrospinal fluid in relatively high concentrations, they were administered intraventricularly as well as systemically. Most patients received methicillin (14 cases) or cephalothin (8 cases) by both routes for two weeks. Of 16 patients treated in this way without shunt removal, 9 were cured and 7 were not. These 7 were subsequently cured after shunt removal. The remaining 6 patients were treated with shunt removal in addition to antibiotics and all were cured.

Shurtleff *et al.* (1974) treated 66 cases of ventriculo–atrial shunt infection due to coagulase-negative staphylococci. Drugs used for treatment were chosen on the basis of *in vitro* sensitivity tests and the expectation of bactericidal blood levels at normal systemic dosage. A variety of antibiotics were used, and the cases were divided into six groups. The first group of 23 were given systemic antibiotics without surgical intervention. Only 2 of these patients were cured, as judged by follow-up for six months with negative blood and ventricular or shunt fluid cultures. In the second group of 14 patients, systemic antibiotics were administered and the shunt system was only partially removed, leaving part of the original shunt in place. There were 3 cures in this group. The third group consisted of 12 patients who had their shunts completely replaced during a course of systemic antibiotics. All 12 of these patients were cured of their shunt infection. In a similar group of 7 patients who had complete shunt replacement with both systemic and intraventricular antibiotics; again all patients were cured. The fifth group of 4 patients received antibiotics systemically and by injection into the shunt, but without any surgical intervention; none were cured. The sixth group of 6 patients received systemic and intraventricular drugs only, again without surgical intervention, and only 3 were cured.

Schoenbaum, Gardner and Shillito (1975) reported results of surgical and non-surgical treatment in 94 cases. Sixty per cent of the infections were due to coagulase-negative staphylococci, and the remainder were mainly due to *Staphylococcus aureus* with some

Gram-negative rods. The antibiotics used varied widely. Forty-eight had ventriculo–atrial shunts, 19 had ventriculoperitoneal shunts and 13 had ventriculo–ureteral shunts. Thirty-six per cent of infections in this last group were due to Gram-negative rods.

Twenty-eight patients with ventriculo–atrial shunts were given systemic drugs without surgery, and 5 were cured, whereas 13 of the 17 patients whose shunts were revised in addition to receiving systemic antibiotics were cured. Neither of the two patients with ventriculoperitoneal shunts who had no revision were cured by drugs alone, but 14 of the 16 who had drugs and shunt revision were cured. In those with a ventriculo–ureteral shunt, 8 out of 13 were cured by drugs alone and 5 out of 8 were cured using drugs together with shunt revision. Only systemic antibiotics were used, no patient in this series receiving them by the intraventricular route.

Luthardt (1970) treated 18 patients with ventriculo–atrial shunt infections non-surgically with antibiotics administered systemically and into the shunt. Nine cases were due to coagulase-negative staphylococci, 8 to *Staphylococcus aureus* and one to 'Achromobacter'. The antibiotics used were those considered appropriate for each organism, but they were not identified. The course of treatment lasted for four to six weeks. Only one patient out of 18 treated was cured.

O'Brien *et al.* (1979) described the results of treatment of 39 cases of shunt infection. No distinction was made between ventriculo–atrial and ventriculoperitoneal shunts. Twenty-three cases were due to coagulase-negative staphylococci and the patients were divided into four groups. The first group consisted of 6 patients who were asymptomatic but whose routine cultures obtained during shunt revision grew coagulase-negative staphylococci. These 6 patients were all treated with intravenous antibiotics without further revision, and were considered cured.

However, in the absence of further information the diagnosis of infection in this group must remain in doubt, as coagulase-negative staphylococci may be recovered from removed shunts in the absence of infection if the method of examination is not carefully designed to avoid this (Bayston *et al.*, 1983). All other patients in the remaining groups were symptomatic.

The second group of 5 patients did not undergo shunt revision but were given intravenous and intraventricular antibiotics. In contrast to the experience of other workers, O'Brien achieved a cure in all 5 of these, though the criteria for cure are not defined. Two of these cases were due to *Propionibacterium sp.*, 1 to *Klebsiella sp.*, one to a coagulase-negative staphylococcus and 1 to an unidentified organism. Intravenous and intraventricular antibiotics were combined with shunt removal and immediate replacement in the third group of 19 patients. Fifteen of these were cured of their infections. The remaining 4 patients, who all developed infections in their new shunts, were treated successfully by shunt removal, with delayed replacement after clearing of the infection. The 9 patients in the fourth group were all treated in this way and all were cured.

In consideration of the conflicting views regarding the best way of treating shunt infections, particularly as to whether shunt removal was necessary, James *et al.* (1980) carried out a prospective randomized trial involving 30 patients, all with ventriculoperitoneal shunts. Identification of the causative organisms and determination of their antibiotic sensitivities was carried out by aspiration of the shunt (Myers and Schoenbaum, 1975). None of the patients had wound infections or sepsis in other sites. Sixteen shunts were colonized with coagulase-negative staphylococci and 3 with *Staphylococcus aureus*. A further 5 were mixed infections involving *Streptococcus pyogenes*, *Pseudomonas aeruginosa*, *Corynebacterium spp.*, coliforms, coagulase-negative staphylococci and *Staphylococcus aureus*. One wonders whether at least one of these mixed infections especially those involving coliforms were the result of visceral perforation by the distal catheter (Brook *et al.*, 1977).

A variety of antibiotics were used, and the criteria for cure included negative shunt aspirations two days and one to two months after stopping treatment. The follow-up time was between two months and two years with an average of 23 months. Ten patients were randomly assigned to each of three treatment groups. Patients in Group A had their shunts removed, external ventricular drainage being necessary in 5 cases. Intravenous antibiotics were given, as well as intraventricular antibiotics for at least seven days. All patients in this group were cured of their infections.

Patients in Group B had their shunts removed and immediate insertion of a new one during the same operation. They all received antibiotics through the new shunt reservoir for at least three weeks. Nine of these patients were cured of their infections, the tenth producing a positive cerebrospinal fluid culture with a strain of coagulase-negative staphylococcus having a similar antibiogram to the strain originally causing the infection. This patient was treated again, this time successfully, according to the Group A protocol using external ventricular drainage.

Another patient in Group B required revision after completion of the course of treatment because of distal catheter obstruction. The new shunt was clear of infection and was revised to a ventriculo–atrial shunt.

The patients in Group C did not have their shunts removed but received antibiotics into the shunt reservoir for at least two weeks and intravenously for three weeks. Only 3 of these patients were cured of their shunt infections. Five of the remainder were eventually cured after shunt removal and external drainage as in Group A. The remaining 2 patients in Group C died despite this course of action. One was secondarily infected with *Escherichia coli* and *Pseudomonas* and the other had mechanical problems with the drainage device. Secondary infection also occurred in 1 patient in Group A but this was apparently controlled.

Apart from the obviously superior results with shunt removal, particularly in Group A, and the worrying mortality in Group C, a further factor was found to favour this course of action. Group A patients spent an average of 24 days in hospital, Group B 33 days, and Group C 47 days. While it may be argued that the numbers in this study are small, some of the disadvantages of larger studies are nevertheless overcome. The study was not multicentric, the trial was completed within the relatively short period of four years, and it was prospective. The authors say that 'intraventricular' drugs were administered via the shunt reservoir, but in certain types of shunting device it is difficult to ensure that they enter the ventricular system rather than escaping down the shunt. Nevertheless, the measured drug levels in the ventricular fluid in the treatment failures in Group C did not differ from the successes and there was only one case in each subgroup where the drug levels could be considered to be therapeutic on the basis of the minimum inhibitory concentration for the infecting organism. The obvious conclusion drawn by James *et al.* was that in only rare situations should treatment without shunt removal be attempted.

The use of intraventricular antibiotics with shunt removal in shunt infections due to Gram-negative bacteria has been reported. Olsen, Grotte and Nordbring (1977) described a child with a ventriculo-peritoneal shunt who developed ventriculitis due to *Pseudomonas aeruginosa* at the age of 8 months. Gentamicin was administered, both intramuscularly and intraventricularly, and the shunt was removed. The cerebrospinal fluid eventually became sterile after more than two weeks and a new shunt was subsequently inserted uneventfully. An interesting aspect of this case is the high cerebrospinal fluid levels of gentamicin achieved. An intraventricular dose of 3 mg daily gave levels of 25–35 mg/l 24 hours after injection, and on one occasion this rose to 76 mg/l. Intraventricular gentamicin was administered daily for a total of 35 days with no evidence of toxicity or irritation. Other workers have reported very high cerebrospinal fluid gentamicin levels after intraventricular administration with no ill effects (Lorber, Rhoton and Mellinger, 1970; Kourtopoulos and Holm, 1976). Indeed, in Olsen's case the cerebrospinal fluid became sterile for the first time immediately following the high trough level of 76 mg/l (but see Welch, 1977 and Chapter 6).

Katz, Rapp and Walsh (1980) reported a 4-month-old girl with a ventriculoperitoneal shunt which was infected with *Enterobacter cloacae*. She was treated with intravenous carbenicillin and intraventricular gentamicin 2 mg daily. The intraventricular dose was progressively increased to 6 mg daily. The trough gentamicin levels in the cerebrospinal fluid were 1.7 mg/l for 2 mg, and 19.6 mg/l for 6 mg. The infection in this patient was eradicated without shunt removal, but a secondary shunt infection with *Klebsiella pneumoniae*, possibly due to intraventricular injections, was followed by blockage of the distal catheter. Gram-negative rods may be easier than staphylococci to eradicate from shunts with antibiotics alone, as there is reason to believe that they are often not capable of attaching themselves to the silicone rubber in the same way as staphylococci. While some Gram-negative rods are certainly capable of attachment to polymers (Sugarman, 1982; Marrie, Noble and Costerton, 1983) they do not appear to surround themselves with a dense matrix as in the case of coagulase-negative staphylococci. This may explain the successful non-surgical treatment by Olsen and Katz.

5.2   SHUNT REMOVAL

In Shurtleff's cases, where several groups of patients were given systemic or intraventricular antibiotics or both, with and without shunt removal, satisfactory cure rates were achieved only where the infected shunt was completely removed, in conjunction with systemic antibiotics (Groups 3 and 4).

Similarly, Schoenbaum's findings indicate that patients who have their infected shunts completely removed have a much better chance of cure. Luthardt's lack of success with antibiotics alone emphasizes this, as does Callaghan's failure to eradicate the infection in his patients without shunt removal even when methicillin was administered intraventricularly for several weeks.

One cannot escape the obvious conclusion, so amply demonstrated by James *et al.* (1980), that the method of choice for treatment of shunt infection is complete surgical removal of the shunt. However, shunt removal is not without its disadvantages. If the placement of a new shunt is delayed, and external ventricular drainage is not instituted, then problems may be encountered with control of cerebrospinal fluid pressure. Frequent ventricular taps may be used, but these do not give good control and may lead to porencephalic cysts and introduction of micro-organisms into the ventricles. If external ventricular drainage is used there is a risk of ventriculitis due to contaminating organisms ascending the drainage tube. If a three-way tap is included in the system, this represents a considerable risk of contamination and consequent secondary ventriculitis. Also, if the original infection is not completely eradicated before placement of the new shunt, recurrence of shunt infection may result.

In addition, some patients are unfortunate enough to be cured of their shunt infection by shunt removal, only to contract a different infection in their new shunt. Four of O'Brien's cases fell into this group. These patients may represent an even greater therapeutic problem as the second infection is likely to be due to an organism which is more resistant to antibiotics than the first one due to the antibiotic treatment for the first infection.

There is strong evidence that, in the case of infections with *Haemophilus influenzae*, neisseria and pneumococci, cure can be achieved without surgical intervention. Indeed, in all ill patients an operation might well worsen their chances of recovery. Shurtleff, Foltz and Christie (1971) remarked that standard parenteral antibiotic therapy had produced a complete cure in their case of Haemophilus meningitis. Sells, Shurtleff and Loesser (1977) also described a similar successful case, though this might have been the same patient as Shurtleff's.

Rennels and Wald (1980) describe 4 cases of *Haemophilus influenzae* meningitis, 3 of whom were treated successfully with intravenous chloramphenicol 100 mg/kg/day for ten to sixteen days. One of these was a 4-year-old child with histiocytosis X. Patriarca and Lauer (1980) treated 2 cases but here systemic and intraventricular ampicillin was used in both cases, with intravenous chloramphenicol additionally in the second. The first child required surgery for a disconnection of the proximal part of the shunt, but only part of the original shunt was removed. This patient recovered. The second patient, however, had persistently positive cerebrospinal fluid cultures for *Haemophilus influenzae* despite back titrations showing bactericidal activity in the cerebrospinal fluid to a dilution of 256, and the shunt was revised. After initial recovery, the patient relapsed 51 days after admission with positive cultures for Haemophilus, but this time complete cure was achieved using the same regimen as previously but without further surgery.

Two different regimens were used in two reported cases (Stern, Bayston and Hayward, 1988). In the first, the shunt was not removed and chloramphenicol was given with satisfactory result. In the second, the shunt was exteriorized and cefuroxime was given. After five days the shunt, with the exception of the ventricular catheter, was removed and a new one inserted using the remaining upper catheter. The infection relapsed within days requiring complete removal of the new shunt and upper catheter and a two-week course of cefuroxime. It is felt that chloramphenicol should have been used in the second case, without shunt surgery.

Two cases of meningococcal meningitis are recorded (Schoenbaum, Gardner and Shillito, 1975; cited by Noble and Cooper, 1977; Leggiadro, Atluru and Katz, 1984). The first patient was cured without recourse to surgery, though the details of treatment are not given. The second patient was an 11-month-old infant with two ventriculoperitoneal shunts, who had a rash and fever. *Neisseria meningitidis* was isolated from the cerebrospinal fluid, and he was treated non-surgically with intravenous penicillin 250 000 units/kg/day for two weeks with rapid and complete recovery.

A further case of gonococcal meningitis, reported by Noble and Cooper (1977), involved a 21-year-old woman who had had a spontaneous abortion six weeks before admission. She had a ventriculoperitoneal shunt for hydrocephalus of unknown cause. One week before admission she had neck stiffness and fever, along with purulent vaginal discharge. *Neisseria gonorrhoeae* was isolated from her cerebrospinal fluid and she was given 4 mega units of penicillin intravenously four-hourly for 12 days. Her symptoms resolved rapidly and she made a complete recovery. There is also evidence that pneumococcal meningitis in shunted patients can also be treated without shunt removal, as in 2 cases in our experience. One might expect that the presence of a ventriculo–atrial shunt in a patient with meningitis due to haemophilus, gonococcus or meningococcus would lead to a more severe illness with uncontrollable septicaemia. In fact, this was not the case with Schoenbaum's and Sell's cases. Similarly, one would expect peritonitis to be a serious problem in the management of such patients with ventriculoperitoneal shunts, but again this does not seem to be so. Indeed, there was not even any evidence of distal shunt occlusion which is so often found in ventriculoperitoneal shunt infections with staphylococci. It appears that such cases can safely be managed non-surgically, using intravenous chloramphenicol for haemophilus and intravenous penicillin for the neisseria and pneumococci.

5.3   SHUNT REMOVAL AND IMMEDIATE RESHUNTING

The risks associated with the intervening period between removal of an infected shunt and insertion of a new one have led to attempts to insert a new shunt at the same operation as that to remove the infected one. Nicholas, Kamal and Eckstein (1970) compared the results of treatment in one group of 31 patients who had delayed shunt replacement with another group of 27 patients who had a new shunt inserted at the operation for shunt removal. All patients had Holter ventriculo–atrial shunts. In the delayed method a course of an antibiotic to which the infecting organism was susceptible *in vitro* was begun, and the infected shunt was removed. The antibiotics were given intrathecally if the ventricular system was infected, and pressure was controlled as necessary by ventricular taps. After five days the drugs were stopped and blood and cerebrospinal fluid were cultured. If results were negative a new ventriculo–atrial shunt was inserted. In the immediate replacement method antibiotics were begun 24 hours before surgery. The shunt was removed and a large bolus of a suitable antibiotic was given intravenously. After a delay of at least 20 minutes the new shunt was inserted into the same vein, and the antibiotics were continued for at least five days postoperatively. In the delayed group there were 8 failures out of 31, and in the immediate replacement group there were 6 failures out of 23, making the failure rate in each group 26%.

While immediate replacement would avoid the risks of secondary sepsis associated with external drainage or ventricular taps, it is certainly not without its problems. As Nicholas *et al.* state, if there are organisms in the cerebrospinal fluid, rather than being confined to the shunt, they cannot possibly be cleared by one intravenous injection of an antibiotic. In addition, the same vein cannot often be used due to calcification, adhesion of the catheter, venous occlusion and contamination from the previous shunt. These problems were encountered in Nicholas's patients. The method is more likely to succeed if intraventricular, as well as intravenous antibiotics are used but again it is doubtful whether one peroperative intraventricular injection would have any effect on established ventriculitis.

An alternative method is that suggested by Forrest (personal communication, 1986). First, specimens of cerebrospinal fluid are taken from the ventricle and the valve chamber for culture. If both grow organisms the shunt is exteriorized and appropriate antimicrobials are given both intravenously and intraventricularly for ten days. If the ventricular fluid shows a normal cell count and no growth then the infected shunt is removed and a new one replaced at the same operation. After full head shaving and preparation, the whole shunt is withdrawn through a small scalp incision. With foreknowledge of the infecting organism, a suitable antimicrobial is then injected intravenously, and a waterproof dressing is used to cover the wound. All instruments and drapes are removed from the operating area and surgeons and nurses re-scrub and re-gown. The patient's head is turned to the opposite side. The head is re-prepared and, using a new set of instruments, a new shunt is inserted into a previously unused site. Aseptic and antiseptic technique used is that discussed in Chapter 6, an important component of which may be the introduction of antimicrobial into the shunt and the ventricle and down the vein if the venous route is used.

This technique takes into account the possibility of infection in the ventricular cerebrospinal fluid and is used only where the cerebrospinal fluid is shown to be uninfected. In addition, a different site is used for the for new shunt, rather than inserting it into the existing site as Nicholas recommends.

Despite shunt removal and a variety of antibiotics, in a minority of cases ventriculitis persists. This, along with the problems previously mentioned, means that shunt removal may not be as successful as it at first promises to be. In addition, technical difficulties such as placement of the proximal catheter and the associated prospect of exchanging a shunt which is infected but functioning for one which, while free of infection, fails to give satisfactory pressure control, lead to repeated attempts to eradicate the infection without removal of the shunt.

5.4 ANTIMICROBIALS

The type of antibiotic, its antibacterial spectrum *in vitro*, its known effectiveness *in vivo*, and its pharmacokinetics are sometimes not fully considered in the important and often complicated field of shunt infections. As most shunt infections are caused by staphylococci, those antibiotics known to be effective in infections due to these organisms in other sites are often used. These include oxacillin, cloxacillin or methicillin, cefuroxime, fusidic acid, erythromycin, lincomycin or clindamycin, and vancomycin. These drugs are almost invariably given intravenously.

Many shunt infections are due to organisms which do not provoke a vigorous inflammatory response to the cerebral ventricular system, and ventriculitis is commonly absent in patients with shunt infections in some centres (Callaghan, Cohen and Stewart, 1961; Cohen and Callaghan, 1961; Schimke *et al.*, 1961; Bruce *et al.*, 1963; Perrin and McLaurin, 1967; Stickler *et al.*, 1968; Rames *et al.*, 1970; Bayston and Spitz, 1978) with a consequent lack of inflammation of the 'blood–CSF barrier'. In such situations these drugs do not appear in the cerebrospinal fluid in therapeutic quantities.

There is also an active transport system out of the cerebrospinal fluid compartment (Hieber and Nelson, 1977) responsible for excretion of those drugs which are based on the penicillin nucleus so that even if these drugs are given intraventricularly, their levels may not remain in the therapeutic range for long enough to be effective. This may explain the failure of methicillin in Callaghan's cases, even when it was administered intraventricularly for very long periods. In addition, the presence of inflammation of the 'blood–CSF' not only increases entry of these, and most other, drugs into the cerebrospinal fluid but also decreases the rate of efflux due to the transport system. However, the rate of efflux increases rapidly as the inflammation resolves (Spector and Lorenzo, 1974). This leads to a common situation in which the ventriculitis is cured but the patient's condition deteriorates on stopping treatment due to persistence of colonization in the shunt.

In those cases where antibiotics were administered systemically rather than by the intraventricular route, the failure rate has been high. In addition to the cases described by Callaghan, Cohen and Stewart (1961) where intravenously administered methicillin could not be detected in the cerebrospinal fluid, only 5 of the 37 patients reported by Shurtleff *et al.* (1974) who received intravenous anti-biotics alone in the absence of complete shunt removal were cured, though cerebrospinal fluid levels were not stated. Similarly, only 1 of Luthardt's (1970) 18 cases and 5 of Schoenbaum's (1975) 30 cases of ventriculo–atrial or ventriculoperitoneal shunt infection in which systemic antibiotics alone were used were cured. These reports reflect the experience of others, published and unpublished.

The author has recently measured cerebrospinal fluid cefuroxime levels in 7 patients, 6 of whom had shunt infections, who were receiving the drug intravenously. Therapeutic levels were detected in only 1 patient, this being a child with no evidence of infection but who had an external drain to control pressure due to effusion following intraventricular haemorrhage.

It is interesting to note that excretion of beta-lactam drugs from the cerebrospinal fluid can be considerably reduced by the use of *p*-(dipropylsulphamoyl)-benzoic acid (probenecid) (Spector and Lorenzo, 1974). Unfortunately, this compound also competes with beta-lactam drugs for entry into the cerebrospinal fluid, and the sum of these two effects is a lowering of the drug levels, at least in so far as the brain is concerned (Fishman, 1966). In addition, the excretion of some of the newer cephalosporins is unaffected by probenecid (Luthy *et al.*, 1981).

Comparison of results in O'Brien's (1979) Groups I and II suggests at first sight that both surgery and intraventricular antibiotics may be unnecessary as all patients in these two groups were apparently cured and only those in Group II received intraventricular drugs. However, mention has already been made of the possibly doubtful diagnosis in Group I. Furthermore, if intravenous drugs alone were so successful one would expect a 100% cure rate in Group III, where drugs given by both intravenous and intraventricular routes were combined with surgery. This may actually have been so, as the 4 'recurrences' in this group were probably not treatment failures but new infections. In that case, the cure rate in all groups is 100%, even where only systemic antibiotics were used. These findings are not consistent with those of other authors, and unfortunately the lack of details regarding diagnosis and follow-up, and of criteria for cure, do not allow further evaluation of this paper.

Other drugs must be introduced directly into the ventricular system if successful treatment is to be achieved without shunt removal.

5.5 CELL-WALL-ACTIVE ANTIMICROBIALS

Methicillin has been widely used in North America, and occasionally in Great Britain. Other cell-wall-active (CWA) drugs such as ampicillin, cloxacillin, oxacillin or cefuroxime have also been used extensively to treat shunt infections, but where the shunt has not been removed the treatment has usually failed even when they have been given intraventricularly. The cases reported by Callaghan, Cohen and Stewart (1961), in which methicillin was used unsuccessfully have been discussed already. James *et al.* (1980) used a variety of antibiotics, but in their Group C, patients received systemic and intraventricular CWA antibiotics (ampicillin, methicillin or cephalothin) without surgery, with poor results. When this author reviewed results of non-surgical treatment with antibiotics alone it was found that of 7 patients with shunt infections due to coagulase-negative staphylococci who received systemic cloxacillin alone, none were cured, and the same poor results were also obtained with this antibiotic in 4 patients who received it intraventricularly but not systemically, as well as in 3 patients who received it by both routes (Bayston and Rickwood, 1981).

An important factor to consider here is the ability of CWA drugs to kill staphylococci. Traditionally, penicillin and therefore the semi-synthetic and synthetic CWA drugs, have been regarded as bactericidal antibiotics. The meaning of this term in the absence of qualification is now often questioned, and the same bactericidal drug may be bacteriostatic in lower concentration (Nishino and Nakazawa, 1976). Also, CWA drugs act only upon actively growing cells (Hartmann, Holtje and Schwarz, 1972), and it is likely that, at least in shunts, the colonizing bacteria are growing only slowly if at all in some situations. Osmolality also has an effect on the action of CWA drugs *in vitro* (Greenwood and O'Grady, 1972; Bayston and Swinden, 1981) and in some cases *in vivo* (Strominger and Tipper, 1965), in that the higher the osmolality the less readily the bacteria whose cell walls have been damaged will lyse. All these factors, along with the nature of the microcolonies in colonized shunts, in which extracellular slime may also offer protection to the organisms (see Chapter 2) probably contribute to the explanation of generally poor results using CWA drugs.

5.6   INTRAVENTRICULAR ANTIMICROBIALS

Intraventricular antimicrobials are sometimes unnecessary following removal of an infected shunt. The reason for this in those cases where ventriculitis is not present is self-evident. In cases where there is ventriculitis, this sometimes clears satisfactorily in the absence of a shunt and with the use of systemic antibiotics alone. Indeed, in some cases it has resolved spontaneously before therapy can be instituted. While the cerebrospinal fluid levels achieved with systemic drugs in the presence of even low-grade inflammation of the 'blood–CSF barrier' are apparently sometimes sufficient to eradicate ventriculitis due to coagulase-negative staphylococci or coryneforms in these circumstances, much higher concentrations are obviously necessary to eradicate infection from the shunt catheters.

Intraventricular administration is therefore essential if sufficient antibiotic is to reach the organisms colonizing the shunt, and this route must be used if attempts to eradicate the infection without removing the shunt are to have any chance of success. In the author's view, intraventricular therapy is also desirable even after shunt removal. One must always remember too that, in ventriculoperitoneal shunts, there is infection of the peritoneal cavity, and though this does not necessarily amount to peritonitis in a traditional sense, the administration of a suitable systemic antibiotic in addition to the intraventricular drugs is essential to treat the peritoneal infection.

5.7   ORAL AND SYSTEMIC ANTIMICROBIALS

A limited number of orally or systemically administered antimicrobials will produce therapeutic levels in the cerebrospinal fluid of normal individuals, and therefore their usefulness in the treatment of shunt infections should be considered. These drugs are trimethoprim, rifampicin, some sulphonamides, chloramphenicol and possibly ceftriaxone. The last is a relatively new beta-lactam antibiotic

which gives high cerebrospinal fluid levels because of the exception-
ally high and sustained blood levels on normal dosage. However,
while it has been used successfully in cases of meningitis (Del Rio
et al., 1982) it has been used without effect to treat shunt infections
(Chonmaitree *et al.*, 1984) and bacteriological studies suggest that it
is not likely to have very high activity against staphylococci.

Chloramphenicol

Chloramphenicol is used a great deal for neurosurgical infections
because of its broad spectrum and the fact that therapeutic quantities
are usually detectable even in 'normal' cerebrospinal fluid after
appropriate systemic and even oral dosage. While many strains of
staphylococci are sensitive *in vitro*, therapeutic results are usually
disappointing in shunt infections due to these organisms. Shurtleff
et al. (1974) obtained 1 cure in 7 patients who were treated with
chloramphenicol without shunt removal. Visconti and Peters (1979)
reported a case of ventriculoperitoneal shunt infection due to coagulase-negative staphylococci where the organism was sensitive to
chloramphenicol, but systemic treatment with this drug failed to
clear the infection, resulting in shunt removal. Ring *et al.* (1979)
reported 2 cases of shunt infection with coagulase-negative staphylococci where the ventricular infection persisted after shunt removal
during treatment with chloramphenicol, combined in 1 case with
nafcillin and in another with methicillin. The one case in the author's
series (Bayston and Rickwood, 1981), a patient with a ventriculo–
atrial shunt colonized by a strain of coagulase-negative staphylococci
which was sensitive to the drug *in vitro*, was treated with intramuscular and intraventricular chloramphenicol without effect.

The author has also seen a patient with a ventriculoperitoneal
shunt colonized by a susceptible strain of coagulase-negative staphylococcus, who also had shunt nephritis, treated with chloramphenicol. The patient rapidly became apyrexial but the
nephropathy progressed and caused death some months later. The
shunt was still heavily colonized when aspirated just prior to death.

Failure of chloramphenicol in the presence of a shunt may be
related to its mode of action on bacteria coupled with the known
nature of the microcolonies in the shunt. Chloramphenicol exerts its
antibacterial effect by binding to the 50S subunit of the bacterial
ribosome, thus preventing the synthesis of peptide chains. This
binding is reversible, and after exposure to the drug the partially-

formed peptide chains can then be completed and protein synthesis can proceed (Green, Cameron and Julian, 1975). With sustained high drug levels, bacterial death occurs, but in most cases the levels will fluctuate between doses. Another factor is the growth phase of the target organisms (Gupta, 1975). Slowly dividing cells are much less susceptible to the drug, and in microcolonies in shunts the majority of organisms seem to be in the stationary phase. A further probable factor is the limited penetration of the microcolonies due to the extracellular matrix (see Chapter 2).

Co-trimoxazole

Two other compounds which penetrate well into the cerebrospinal fluid are trimethoprim and sulphamethoxazole which are sold together as co-trimoxazole. Bayston and Rickwood (1981) found that 2 of 4 cases of ventriculoperitoneal shunt colonization due to co-agulase-negative staphylococci were cured when oral co-trimoxazole was used alone without shunt removal. One of the failures was associated with resistance to the drug and the other was probably due to curtailment of the drug treatment when the shunt blocked soon after it began. In addition, 4 of 7 cases of ventriculo–atrial shunt colonization due to this group of organisms were cured without shunt removal when oral co-trimoxazole was used, though all 7 were given gentamicin intraventricularly in addition. One of the failures involved a gentamicin-resistant strain, and 2 were patients whose Holter shunts did not incorporate a reservoir, necessitating injection of the gentamicin into the shunt pumping chamber. In the author's experience, this mode of administration is a further factor leading to failure, and this is borne out by other studies (Shurtleff *et al.*, 1974). Co-trimoxazole has a wide antibacterial spectrum though an appreciable number of strains show resistance *in vitro*. The attractions of this combination include the synergy which should result from the sequential blockade of purine synthesis by first sulphamethoxazole and then trimethoprim. However, such synergy is not so pronounced *in vivo* (Darrell, Garrod and Waterworth, 1968) and the clinical relevance of *in vitro* synergy has been questioned (Brumfitt and Pursell, 1972; Kasanen *et al.*, 1974). Differential accumulation into various sites in the body also occurs, so that even if the combination is administered in the proportions most likely to lead to synergy, the two drugs are often present at the site of infection in entirely different proportions (Stamey and Condy, 1975).

In addition, on several occasions rashes have been encountered in patients receiving co-trimoxazole, and these have resolved rapidly on changing to trimethoprim. The author's normal practice is now to use trimethoprim initially intravenously without sulphamethoxazole.

Rifampicin

Rifampicin could until recently only be given orally, but even so in many patients therapeutic cerebrospinal fluid levels are achieved in the presence of an intact, uninflamed 'blood–CSF barrier'. Indeed, Wake, Humphrey and Walker (1980) described a patient with only 32 cm of small bowel who had satisfactory serum rifampicin levels after oral therapy, though in cases of frank malabsorption syndrome blood levels are likely to be very variable (Wasson and Harris, 1976).

The intravenous preparation is now available and has proved safe in use (Acocella *et al.*, 1977; Nitti *et al.*, 1977; Kissling, Bergamini and Xilinas, 1982) though in the case of both the oral and the intravenous routes there is early elevation of liver enzymes due to stimulation of hepatocytic activity. The simultaneous administration of other drugs which are metabolized by the liver should be avoided if possible. It is also noteworthy that staff administering or dispensing rifampicin have been known to experience allergic effects (Anker and Bang, 1981).

Both Nitti *et al.* (1977) and Wake, Humphrey and Walker (1980) have found little difference in blood levels when rifampicin is given orally or intravenously, but poor cerebrospinal fluid levels have sometimes been seen in patients on oral therapy. Unfortunately, the serum levels were not simultaneously measured but it is likely that they were unsatisfactorily low, and the intravenous preparation has since been found to be more reliable in producing therapeutic cerebrospinal fluid levels.

Rifampicin inhibits bacterial protein synthesis by binding to RNA polymerase. The drug is highly lipid soluble and has been shown to concentrate inside polymorphonuclear leucocytes and to kill phagocytosed staphylococci (Mandell, 1973; Ezer and Soothill, 1974). Almost all strains of coagulase-negative staphylococci isolated by the author from the skin surfaces of patients undergoing shunt surgery have been sensitive to rifampicin *in vitro*, with the notable exception of a strain from a patient receiving rifampicin for tuberculosis, and the very good antistaphylococcal activity of this drug has been reported by others (Sabath, Garner and Wilcox, 1976). However, resistance develops rapidly when staphylococci are exposed to the drug *in vitro* (Archer, Tenenbaum and Haywood, 1978), and unless combination therapy is used, this also occurs *in vivo* (Mandell and Moorman, 1980). Rifampicin combined with another drug has been used to treat shunt infections caused by coagulase-negative staphylococci (Archer, Tenenbaum and Haywood, 1978; Ring *et al.*, 1979), and meningitis due to enterococci (Ryan *et al.*, 1980).

In one of Archer's cases, a 17-year-old girl with a ventriculoperitoneal shunt infection due to coagulase-negative staphylococcus, a variety of antibiotics had been administered, including intraventricular gentamicin and intravenous vancomycin, without effect. Rifampicin, given in a single oral dose of 600 mg daily, was added to a regimen consisting of the above two drugs and dramatic clinical and bacteriological improvement ensued, followed by complete recovery though only after removal of the infected shunt.

Two cases were reported by Ring. One was a 24-day-old girl and the other was a 4½-month-old boy. Both had ventriculoperitoneal shunts which were infected with coagulase-negative staphylococci and these were removed. Despite treatment with chloramphenicol and nafcillin in the first case and chloramphenicol and methicillin in the second, the ventricular infections were not eradicated. In the first case the treatment was changed to intravenous vancomycin and oral rifampicin and in the second oral rifampicin was added to the existing treatment regimen. In both cases rapid clinical and bacteriological recovery followed and both patients were successfully reshunted.

Rifampicin has been used successfully in staphylococcal infections when combined with a variety of drugs, and its use in conjunction with trimethoprim has been reported (Grüneberg, Emmerson and Ridgway, 1984).

5.8 AMINOGLYCOSIDES

The aminoglycosides have proved to be a very useful group of drugs for the treatment of infections, including meningitis, due to a variety of bacteria over many years. They exert their bactericidal effect by binding to the bacterial ribosomes, thus interfering with protein synthesis. Because of the consequent mis-coding of m-RNA, non-functional proteins are produced. Aminoglycosides in current use systemically are streptomycin, kanamycin, gentamicin, tobramycin, amikacin and netilmicin.

One of the disadvantages of the aminoglycosides is the low therapeutic index. Serum drug levels (peak and trough) must be determined at intervals to ensure that therapeutic activity is achieved without excessive levels which can lead to toxicity, affecting the eighth cranial nerve and the kidney.

The degree of toxicity varies from one aminoglycoside to another. Eighth cranial nerve function is compromised by damage to the hair cells of either the cochlea or the vestibule. In the case of deafness the effect may not be total hearing loss, as damage to the inner cochlear hair cells only, for instance, will allow hearing but will not enable discrimination between similar sounds. While all aminoglycosides can be said to be both ototoxic and nephrotoxic, the proportional effects vary considerably. Streptomycin, while being the least nephrotoxic, may cause vestibular and cochlear damage, as may gentamicin, which also sometimes causes cochlear damage and nephrotoxicity. Amikacin and kanamycin both cause mainly cochlear damage. Netilmicin appears to be less ototoxic, causing less than one-fifth the cochlear damage due to gentamicin, and is less nephrotoxic. Netilmicin would therefore appear to be the aminoglycoside of choice on these grounds.

Another disadvantge of this group of drugs is that they penetrate the cerebrospinal fluid very poorly, and in the absence of florid inflammation there is little likelihood of achieving effective cerebrospinal fluid concentrations. Gentamicin sulphate has been used intraventricularly to treat meningitis (Newman and Holt, 1967; Lorber, Rhoton and Mellinger, 1970; Newman and Holt, 1971; and others), and this route has also been utilized in the treatment of shunt infections (Olsen, Grotte and Nordbring, 1977; Katz, Rapp and Walsh, 1980; Bayston and Rickwood, 1981). The cases described by Olsen and Katz involved Gram-negative rods and the infections were cleared without shunt removal.

In the author's series of 39 coagulase-negative staphylococcus shunt infections in which an attempt was made to clear the infection without shunt removal, 14 patients received intraventricular gentamicin. In 4 cases this was used alone and treatment was unsuccessful. In the remaining 10 cases it was combined with either chloramphenicol, cloxacillin (intraventricular in 1 case) or cotrimoxazole. Only in those cases where co-trimoxazole was used in addition to intraventricular gentamicin was there any success in eradication of the infection. This occurred in 4 out of 7 cases. Two failures were associated with absence of a reservoir, another being ascribed to pre-existing gentamicin resistance in the infecting organism. Of the 4 successful cases, 3 required subsequent shunt revision at four and seven months and two-and-a-half years respectively for blockage, and at the revision the cerebrospinal fluid and shunt were found to be free from bacteria. The fourth child was fit with normal shunt serology after five years.

While this drug regimen might allow retention of a functioning shunt, a possible risk has suggested itself. In 2 cases, treated since the above study, the infection has been successfully eradicated but within four months and six months respectively the patients have presented with ventriculitis due to a mixture of enteric organisms. This was thought to be due to perforation of the bowel by the shunt tubing. A previous infection, though successfully eradicated, may predispose to this by either fixation of the shunt tubing or softening of the enteric lymphoid tissue or both.

There is little evidence that intraventricular administration of aminoglycosides even if it results in high levels in the cerebrospinal fluid, leads to ototoxicity, though, of course, this lack of evidence may merely reflect a lack of investigation. It is none the less worth noting that, in a study by Welch (1977), some evidence of ototoxicity was seen with high intraventricular doses which were also associated with seizures. However, the concentration of the drug in the perilymph is considered to be important. High plasma concentrations lead to high concentrations in the perilymph but high cerebrospinal fluid concentrations in the absence of parenteral administration may not do so.

The existence of direct connections between the subarachnoid space and the perilymph is a subject of debate, and if anatomically present they may not function as such. The evidence suggests that the majority of the perilymph is derived from the plasma and is not an extension of the cerebrospinal fluid.

Also, Hodges *et al.* (1981) studied neurological and pathological changes in rabbits which received gentamicin by ventriculostomy. Both pathological and neurological changes were absent or negligible in animals receiving 0.05 mg/kg/day (approximately 0.1 mg daily) but in two other groups, receiving 0.25 mg/kg/day (approximately 0.5 mg daily) and 0.5 mg/kg/day (approximately 1 mg daily), significant neurological changes appeared during life and at necropsy chemical ventriculitis with macrophage infiltration and gross loss of microvilli and cilia from the ependymal cells was noted. In the two groups with evidence of toxicity, high concentrations of gentamicin in the cerebrospinal fluid, reaching 300 mg/l were found, but most were around 20–60 mg/l.

Apart from possible differences between rabbits and humans in respect of sensitivity of central nervous system tissue to gentamicin, two other considerations should be taken into account. One is that, in humans, daily intraventricular doses in excess of those used in the rabbits have generally resulted in lower cerebrospinal fluid levels (Katz, Rapp andWalsh, 1980). The other is that, even where very high levels of gentamicin have been achieved, there have been no ill effects (Lorber, Rhoton and Mellinger, 1970; Kourtopoulos and Holm, 1976; Olson, Grotte and Nordbring, 1977) with the possible exception of Welch's (1977) cases. However, it would be prudent not to use unreasonably high doses, and 5 mg should serve as a maximum daily dose. This should be decreased where the patient's ventricular volume is known to be low. In addition, one should also bear in mind the risk of underdosage with consequent failure of treatment and increase in risk and severity of neurological damage.

5.9   VANCOMYCIN

With the appearance of multiple-resistant strains of *Staphylococcus aureus*, vancomycin, which has been in intermittent use since 1957, has enjoyed new popularity. This antibiotic, like the related drugs, ristocetin and teicoplanin, is a glycopeptide with a relatively high molecular weight. It is active mainly against Gram-positive bacteria. While no resistant strains of staphylococci have been isolated, some strains of streptococci, particularly enterococci, have been reported to be resistant (Toala, McDonald and Wilcox, 1969; Harwick, Kalmanson and Guze, 1973) though most are susceptible. Coryneforms, including 'JK' groups, listeria and clostridia are also susceptible.

The drug acts by interfering with cell-wall synthesis, binding irreversibly to the newly-synthesized peptide chains at D-alanine. This prevents release of bactoprenol and blocks incorporation of the new glycopeptide into the cell wall (Watanakunakorn, 1981). There is also some evidence that the drug alters the permeability of the cell membrane (Riley, 1970) and that it selectively inhibits RNA synthesis

(Jordan and Inniss, 1959). Perhaps due to these multiple sites of action, L-forms are virtually impossible to produce *in vitro* and are extremely unlikely to be produced as a result of treatment.

Tolerance, a situation where the minimum inhibitory concentration is greatly exceeded by the minimum cidal concentration *in vitro*, has been demonstrated in *Staphylococcus aureus* (Watanakunakorn, 1978) and in *Staphylococcus epidermidis* (Traub, 1981), but there is doubt about the clinical significance of this phenomenon.

Vancomycin is usually administered intravenously, except in cases of enterocolitis when it is given orally. Unfortunately, penetration into the cerebrospinal fluid is poor. In a study of cerebrospinal fluid concentrations after intravenous administration of staphylococcal sepsis, Nolan *et al.* (1980) found that cerebrospinal fluid levels were low and on only 2 occasions exceeded the minimum inhibitory concentration.

Their first patient had been on haemodialysis for two years and had developed a *Staphylococcus aureus* septicaemia from an arteriovenous fistula infection. There was clinical meningism with increased protein level and cell count in the cerebrospinal fluid, though no organisms were isolated. No cerebrospinal fluid shunt was present.

The second patient had received haemodialysis for one year because of chronic glomerulonephritis. She developed coagulase-negative staphylococcal bacteraemia which was subsequently found to be due to a long-standing ventriculo–atrial shunt colonization. Cerebrospinal fluid cell-count and protein were normal though a coagulase-negative staphylococcus was isolated. Interestingly, it appears likely that this second patient was suffering from shunt nephritis, though the authors do not mention this. Certainly, the nephropathy resolved after eradication of the shunt colonization which necessitated removal of the shunt. Both patients received intravenous vancomycin.

Krontz and Strausbaugh (1980) studied the penetration of vancomycin into the cerebrospinal fluid of rabbits with pneumococcal meningitis and found that the levels were higher than those in control, uninfected rabbits, and in most cases in the meningitic group the cultures gave no growth after six hours' therapy. The levels in the uninfected animals were similar to those reported by Nolan *et al.* (1980). The authors also studied the effect of probenecid on the cerebrospinal fluid levels and found that it was without effect.

Intravenous vancomycin has been used successfully to treat

meningitis caused by *Flavobacterium meningosepticum* and by *Staphylococcus aureus* by Hawley and Gump (1973). In both cases other drugs had been used without success. Both patients had elevated cerebrospinal fluid leucocyte counts and protein concentrations, and presumably the inflamed blood–brain barrier was sufficiently permeable to the drug to allow therapeutic quantities to appear in the cerebrospinal fluid in these cases. It must be emphasized that a more vigorous inflammatory response would be expected with the two organisms involved here than with coagulase-negative staphylococci.

Three children with coagulase-negative staphylococcal infections of their ventriculoperitoneal shunts were treated with intravenous vancomycin by Schaad, McCracken and Nelson (1980). The data given suggest a variable but generally moderate inflammatory response, though details are not given. Similarly, the effectiveness in terms of cure are difficult to assess, but the authors state that between 7 and 21% of the serum concentration of vancomycin was found in the cerebrospinal fluid. All 3 patients underwent shunt revision soon after starting the treatment, and in 1 case the cerebrospinal fluid was still infected at this stage.

Visconti and Peters (1979) report 2 cases of shunt-associated ventriculitis due to coagulase-negative staphylococci which were successfully treated with vancomycin. The first patient, a 2-month-old girl with a ventriculo–atrial shunt, had 900 leucocytes/mm^3 in her cerebrospinal fluid, 75% of them neutrophils and a protein content of 76 mg/dl. The shunt was removed and the patient recovered after a ten-day course of intravenous vancomycin.

The second patient was a 2-year-old boy with a ventriculoperitoneal shunt and external drainage. No details of the cellular or protein contents of the cerebrospinal fluid are given. After unsuccessful attempts to treat him with a variety of intravenous and intraventricular drugs, he was given vancomycin both intravenously and intraventricularly (20 mg daily) and his ventriculitis was eradicated. This is probably the first published report of the intraventricular administration of vancomycin.

Ventriculitis due to *Staphylococcus aureus* was treated initially with intravenous vancomycin by Young, Ratner and Clarridge (1981), without success. The infection was eradicated after the addition of intraventricular vancomycin given through an Ommaya reservoir in a daily dose of 20 mg. The organisms failed to grow after six days of this treatment. The concentrations of vancomycin in the cerebrospinal fluid rose from 5 mg/l to 29 mg/l on the introduction of intraventricular therapy.

This form of therapy was also successful in eradicating a persistent coagulase-negative staphylococcal meningitis associated with septi-caemia from a jugular catheter. An unsuccessful attempt to eradicate the infection with intravenous cefotaxime and intraventricular amikacin preceded this.

The patient described by Sutherland *et al.* (1981) had an Ommaya reservoir inserted for treatment of carcinomatous meningitis secondary to ductal carcinoma of the breast. The reservoir became colonized with coagulase-negative staphylococcus and this persisted despite the use of various antimicrobials including intravenous vancomycin. The concentration of vancomycin in the cerebrospinal fluid was found to be 1.2 mg/l, or 3.75% of the serum level. Vanco-mycin was then given into the reservoir in a dose of 75 mcg (*sic*) along with the methotrexate on three occasions and the organisms were eradicated.

The combination of vancomycin with other drugs appears to lead to greater activity in some cases. Though a study by Watanakunakorn and Guerriero (1981) suggests that a combination of vancomycin with rifampicin may be antagonistic against *Staphylococcus aureus in vitro*, this combination has been successfully used in treatment.

Ring *et al.* (1979) reported a patient with persistent coagulase-negative staphylococcal ventriculitis following removal of an in-fected ventriculoperitoneal shunt. This was first treated with chlo-ramphenicol and nafcillin without success, and the regimen was changed to intravenous vancomycin and oral rifampicin. The patient improved promptly and was apyrexial within 24 hours. The infection was eradicated and the patient was successfully re-shunted. Rifampi-cin was also instrumental in the successful treatment of a patient with coagulase-negative staphylococcal ventriculitis following ven-triculoperitoneal shunt infection (Archer, Tenenbaum and Hay-wood, 1978). The patient was treated unsuccessfully with intravenous vancomycin and intraventricular gentamicin but on the addition of oral rifampicin the patient recovered. The cerebrospinal fluid bactericidal reciprocal titres rose with the addition of rifampi-cin from less than 2 to more than 128.

The value of using these two drugs together was further illustrated by Gombert *et al.* (1981), who reported 3 cases treated in this way. In the first case, the infected shunt was removed but the ventriculitis failed to respond to intravenous vancomycin until oral rifampicin was added, when there was prompt bacteriological and clinical recovery followed by successful reshunting. No indication of the ventricular inflammatory response was given, but the cerebrospinal fluid showed a bacteriostatic reciprocal titre of 32 and bactericidal reciprocal titre of 8.

A combination of oral rifampicin with intrathecal and intravenous vancomycin was used by Ryan *et al.* (1980) to treat a 60-year-old man with enterococcal meningitis. Once again, the intraventricular dose was 20 mg daily. Initial treatment was with chloramphenicol, then intravenous vancomycin and gentamicin. Despite there being between 2000 and 5800 leucocytes/mm^3 in the cerebrospinal fluid, measurable drug levels were not achieved and the treatment was changed to vancomycin intravenously and intrathecally. Adequate drug levels were now demonstrated but there was no clinical improvement. Oral rifampicin was added, and the patient's temperature fell and his headache disappeared. The authors state that the enterococcus was inhibited by vancomycin (0.78 mg/l) and by rifampicin (3.12 mg/l) but was not killed by either agent alone *in vitro*.

Because of the variable, but usually poor, penetration of vancomycin into the cerebrospinal fluid in ventriculitis due to coagulase-negative staphylococci, the author and colleagues have administered the drug intraventricularly in 139 episodes. In most cases the daily dose was 20 mg. Fifty of these have been reported (Bayston *et al.*, 1984; Bayston, Hart and Barnicoat, 1987). Their ages ranged from 1 month to 63 years, and their hydrocephalus was associated with a variety of underlying conditions. At the time the infection was diagnosed 28 had ventriculoperitoneal shunts, 12 ventriculo–atrial shunts and in the remainder other routes were used. Forty infections were due to coagulase-negative staphylococci with the remaining 10 due to other Gram-positive organisms. Twenty milligrams of vancomycin daily were given in 38 cases, the others receiving lower doses. A variety of intravenous antimicrobials were used, with rifampicin being given in 23 cases. In a few cases the infected shunt was not removed. In those cases where treatment involved shunt removal, 20 mg of vancomycin daily intraventricularly and another appropriate systemic antimicrobial, 22 of 24 cases were cured with 2 cases showing evidence of cure but becoming lost to long-term follow-up.

Cerebrospinal fluid vancomycin levels reached trough levels of 200–300 mg/l but no toxicity was noted. Where the full dosage is used with shunt removal, reshunting where necessary can be accomplished without risk of relapse in seven to ten days, saving on hospital bed occupancy and decreasing the risk of secondary infection from prolonged external ventricular drainage. Where lower doses were used the success rate was lower. In the 9 cases where the infected shunt was left in place, 5 relapsed on stopping treatment and 1 died from a secondary infection. Only 3, all with ventriculoperitoneal shunts, had their infections eradicated and all required revision for distal end obstruction within four months.

In a series of 20 episodes reported by Swayne, Rampling and Newsom (1987), 20 mg of vancomycin daily were given intraventricularly to adults and 10 mg to children, along with shunt removal. Four patients received no other antimicrobials. One of these relapsed. Thirteen were successfully reshunted and 5 became re-infected. Contrary to the suggestions of Swayne, Rampling and Newsom, this author considers that a systemic antimicrobial in addition to intraventricular vancomycin is advisable (Bayston, 1987) and this is supported by others (Andrew and Waters, 1986). Because of the high success rate and short bed occupancy this regimen is now considered as 'first-line' treatment.

The author saw no evidence of toxicity associated with the use of this regimen, and other workers have also not reported any, with the exception of Sutherland *et al.* (1981). In their case, the patient received 75 μg of intraventricular vancomycin, along with methotrexate, through an Ommaya reservoir. Within minutes the patient experienced a painful throbbing headache which had not occurred when methotrexate alone had been given by this route. The possibility therefore arises of an interaction between the two drugs.

The sensitivity *in vitro* of coagulase-negative staphylococci varies widely from the fully sensitive to those which are totally resistant to almost all antibiotics. Unfortunately, a shift in prevalence towards the highly resistant is now being seen. While intraventricular vancomycin with intravenous rifampicin or another appropriate systemic antimicrobial has proved indispensable in the treatment of shunt-associated ventriculitis, and while resistance is uncommon the use of new treatment regimens may become necessary in future. This may be occasioned by the appearance of resistant strains or the occurrence of infections due to newly-recognized agents. For example, the 'JK' coryneforms will probably increase in importance in implant infections, and though these are at the moment fully susceptible to vancomycin and rifampicin, such drugs as teicoplanin, the new quinolones or perhaps some older rejuvenated antibiotic may find future use.

5.10 RECOMMENDATIONS FOR CURRENT PRACTICE

1. In most cases the shunt should be removed in its entirety as soon as possible after the diagnosis of infection is made, and external ventricular drainage should be instituted. Either a valve should be included in the system, as in the Codman drain, or the continuity of the fluid track should be interrupted by a drip capsule as in the Dow–Corning drain. Both of these devices help to prevent contaminants from ascending to the ventricular system. A competent external drain must be used and it must be properly and carefully managed;

2. Full microbiological examination of samples of cerebrospinal fluid from the ventricular system and from all parts of the removed shunt should be carried out in order to define the site of the infection or colonization. It is particularly important to know whether there is ventricular movement if appropriate chemotherapy is to be used;

3. If no shunt or drainage device is required, so that no access to the ventricular systems is available, rifampicin and another antibiotic, subject to the susceptibility test results, should be given intravenously. Suitable combinations with rifampicin are trimethoprim, fusidic acid or flucloxacillin, though it should be borne in mind that if bacteria are present in the ventricles without a vigorous inflammatory response, fusidic acid and flucloxacillin will not penetrate into the cerebrospinal fluid and in those cases the ventriculitis will persist, requiring intraventricular therapy;

4. If an external drain is used, then intraventricular gentamicin, netilmicin or, preferably, vancomycin should be given alone with intravenous rifampicin or another appropriate antimicrobial. If antibiotic resistance of the organism indicates the intravenous administration of vancomycin, then this should be given by slow infusion to avoid thrombophlebitis and 'red man' syndrome. In some cases, continuity of administration can best be achieved by the use of a central venous catheter;

5. Samples of cerebrospinal fluid should be examined daily by

microscopy and culture and for bacteriostatic and bactericidal titres. The fluid should be withdrawn from the reservoir or upper portion the drain immediately prior to injection of drugs. Duration of treatment must relate to the microbiological results as well as the clinical reponse. No bacteria should be grown from the cerebrospinal fluid beyond day four of treatment. Assuming rapid response, with a return of the cerebrospinal fluid leucocyte count to near-normal levels, and with two or three consecutive daily cultures reported negative after subculture, reshunting, where necessary, should be carried out without delay, and intravenous treatment continued for 24 to 48 hours postoperatively. To wait for a few days while the patient is not on antibiotics before reshunting is tempting fate in the form of drainage-associated sepsis.

6. If the decision is made to attempt to eradicate the infection without shunt removal in a patient with a functioning shunt, then intravenous rifampicin and trimethoprim should be given with either gentamicin or netilmicin or, preferably vancomycin, intraventricularly. If the organism is resistant to trimethoprim this should be omitted. The intraventricular antibiotics should be administered through an integral reservoir, not directly into the shunt at a lower level, as the object is to introduce them into the ventricular system and so ensure a constant perfusion through the shunt. The shunt tubing should be occluded by digital pressure during injection of the drug. Daily cerebrospinal fluid levels should be examined as described above. If the infection is due to pneumococcus, meningococcus, gonococcus, or *Haemophilus influenzae*, then non-surgical treatment offers a good chance of complete success. Intravenous penicillin should be used for meningococcus, gonococcus and pneumococcus and intravenous chloramphenicol for haemophilus.

7. Liver function tests should be performed weekly during rifampicin treatment. These often show transient abnormality but this should not be taken as an indication to stop administration of the drug.

8. The following dosages have been found useful:

Gentamicin intraventricularly	1–5 mg daily
Netilmicin intraventricularly	1–5 mg daily
Vancomycin intraventricularly	20 mg daily

Rifampicin intravenously
 under 12 years   15 mg/kg daily*
 adults   300 mg twice daily
Trimethoprim intravenously
 under 12 years   3 mg/kg thrice daily
 adults   250 mg twice daily

* total dose not to exceed 600 mg daily.

6

PREVENTION OF

SHUNT INFECTIONS

6.1 INTRODUCTION

One reason for studying the aetiology of shunt infections (see Chapter 2) is to guide attempts at their prevention. We now know that virtually all shunt infections, including the so-called 'late' infections, are due to the patient's skin bacteria gaining access to the shunt at operation to insert or revise it. It is not necessary, therefore, to consider the presence of a shunt as a continuing risk of infection if it escapes infection at operation, and therefore not necessary to contemplate long-term antibiotic prophylaxis in shunted patients. Neither does ultra-clean air in the operating theatre offer any advantage over standard positive-pressure theatre ventilation systems in most cases, in view of the known source of offending organisms.

Many attempts at prevention have of course been made by most surgeons who use shunts, but only those reported in the literature can be evaluated. In doing so, it is important to distinguish between genuine shunt colonization, which primarily involves the internal surfaces of the shunt, and infections around the external surface of the system, which really consist of wound infections enhanced by the presence of a foreign body, though internal shunt infection will often lead eventually to external infection if left. In terms of prevention, these two conditions are fundamentally different.

6.2 PREPARATION OF THE PATIENT'S SKIN FOR OPERATION

The object of preparation of the patient's skin before incising it is not to sterilize it. It is to remove any surface organisms which may be contaminating it but which do not belong to the resident flora, and to reduce the numbers of the resident flora as much as possible. A patient who is about to undergo exploration of the biliary tract may have had his skin contaminated with the ward strain of proteus or klebsiella. If these organisms enter the incision then it is possible that they will subsequently give rise to a wound infection. The same is true, of course, for *Staphylococcus aureus*. Such transient surface organisms are usually removed by preoperative skin preparation (though this does not apply to actual skin colonization by *Staphylococcus aureus*), and wound infection due to this cause is relatively uncommon. However, the resident flora of the skin, consisting largely of coryneforms, propionibacteria and coagulase-negative staphylococci, which colonize the hair follicles and glands, are not removed and enter the incision during the operation in large numbers in most cases (Bayston and Lari, 1974; Raahave, 1976). In most operations these organisms are irrelevant and do not cause any problems, though the interesting exception is the occasional stitch abscess, where the stitch behaves as an implant. In operations to insert implants such as shunts, these 'harmless' skin organisms become supremely important, but as has already been pointed out, ordinary methods of skin preparation do not eradicate the resident flora from the deeper layers.

It has been shown (Bayston and Lari, 1974) that, when swabs were taken of the patient's skin before and after routine surgical preparation with aqueous iodine and iodine in alcohol, a relatively large number showed that resident organisms present before preparation had not been removed by the procedure. Also, in many of those where the swab taken after skin preparation grew no organisms, the strains present on the skin prior to preparation appeared in the wound before closure, and were present during insertion and manipulation of the shunt. Though several workers have pointed out that iodine can remove virtually all of intentionally deposited organisms from the skin surface (Gardner and Seddon, 1946; Gardner, 1948; Story, 1952), Price (1951) showed that resident flora below the surface persisted despite application of alcoholic iodine for two minutes. This was confirmed by Saggers and Stewart (1964). A more satisfactory method of skin preparation was therefore sought, as iodine or iodophores alone were clearly unsatisfactory for operations involving implants.

On the assumption that all agents which penetrate deeper into the skin should afford greater protection, dimethylsulphoxide (DMSO) was considered but rejected because it was too penetrative, being known to carry 'passenger' substances with it from the skin surface into the bloodstream. However, a detergent combined with hexachlorophane was found to compare favourably with other agents by Hufnagel, Walter and Howard (1948) and this preparation was marketed as 'Phisohex'. The detergent is a sulphonated ether. The author's studies showed that this preparation sterilized scalp hair on shampooing, the bacteria remaining absent from the hair for several hours, and the same effect was observed when skin was washed using Phisohex. Experiments showed, however, that exogenous recontamination was not prevented during this period, and there was no persisting chemical effect of the antiseptic other than its ability to delay endogenous recolonization of the skin surface due to depletion of the deeper layers (Bayston, 1977). Based on these studies a regimen was devised in which the skin over the proposed incision sites was washed well with Phisohex in the operating theatre and this was then rinsed off and the surface dried with a sterile towel. The area was then painted with alcoholic iodine to prevent exogenous recontamination and to mark the prepared area. This procedure was used in conjunction with other measures. The effect of Phisohex alone was to have been studied but this was not felt worthwhile in view of opposition to its use on the grounds of toxicity. However, Fitzgerald and Connelly (1984) have included the use of 'Phisomed', a similar preparation, in their regimen for skin preparation.

6.3   PREOPERATIVE SCALP SHAVING

Scalp shaving is carried out in a variety of ways. Some surgeons use scissors and an electric razor, while others use traditional or antiseptic shaving cream, and a safety razor. The amount of scalp hair removed also varies. Shaving is sometimes carried out the day before an operation, or it may be done immediately before surgery either on the ward or in the anaesthetic room. The small amount of evidence that exists strongly suggests that shaving more than an hour or two before surgery leads to a heavy bacterial population in association with abrasions and small cuts. This can obviously present an increased risk of surgical infection. There is possibly an increased risk of gross aerial contamination following the use of an electric razor in the anaesthetic room, and while the direction of air flow should keep this out of the operating theatre (but does not always do so) the resulting contamination of the trolley which is usually used to convey the patient to the operating table and of the patient's surgical gown, could conceivably contaminate the theatre environment. A less traumatic, safer and easier method would perhaps be to use the scissors followed by a depilatory cream. Some of these contain substances which have an unacceptable risk of skin hypersensitivity or irritations, but others do not. However, such preparations are rarely used in surgery.

6.4 THE USE OF DRAPES

Surgical drapes are traditionally made from linen or cotton and are totally pervious to blood, sweat, and other fluids. Once wet, they do not prevent passage of bacteria from the underlying skin to their anterior surfaces, and therefore cannot be expected to prevent skin organisms from gaining access to the incision. The use of impervious drapes with an adhesive under-surface ('Steridrape', 3M*) is designed to overcome this problem.

The whole area of the operation, including that surrounding the incision, is covered with the drape after preparation and drying of the skin. Enough is applied to afford a surface from which gloved hands and instruments cannot be contaminated, as with cloth drapes. The cloth drapes are applied first but some distance from the incision and the adhesive drape is then applied to help to hold them in place. The impervious drape must be carefully applied so as to avoid creases as far as possible, as these can act as channels between drape and skin for contaminated fluids. However, despite these precautions the use of such drapes usually has little effect on the rate of wound contamination and therefore on the rate of shunt infection.

Raahave (1976) found no difference in the bacterial load in herniotomy wounds where adhesive plastic drapes had been used compared to controls with conventional drapes, thus confirming the earlier work of Jackson, Pollock and Tindall (1971). Tabara and Forrest (1982) used adhesive drapes (Steridrape) and found that the rate of shunt infection was significantly greater than in another group, simultaneously studied, who received antibiotics. The

*3M Products, Morley Street, Loughborough, Leics., LE11 1EP.

authors suggest that this may be due to the failure of the adhesive drape to remain stuck to the wound edges during the operation, thereby allowing contamination of the wound from this source. This problem has often been observed in the author's hands, as has the accumulation of sweat under the drape, with the occasional consequence of localized detachment and spillage of the sweat into the incision.

6.5 THE USE OF ANTISEPTIC BARRIERS AT WOUND EDGES

Following an appreciation of the importance of the margins of the incision as a source of wound contamination during shunt surgery, we devised a system incorporating the method of skin preparation using Phisohex referred to earlier, but which included antiseptic barriers around the edges of the incision (Bayston, 1977). The barriers took the form of gauze packs soaked in 1% solution of noxythiolin (Geistlich, UK*). This antiseptic has a very broad spectrum and is not toxic or irritant to tissues. Sixty-five wounds packed in this way were studied bacteriologically, along with a further 67 which had an identical procedure with the exception that, instead of noxythiolin, physiological saline was used to soak the packs. Detailed bacteriological studies showed that there was no statistical difference between the two groups in respect of numbers of incisions containing skin organisms or the numbers of organisms in the wounds. The rate of shunt infection in the two groups was similar. Tabara and Forrest (1982) used a similar system of wound packs soaked in noxythiolin and compared the rate of shunt colonization with that in a group where impervious adhesive drapes were used. Again, no difference was found between the rates in the two groups. In this study, the shunt was irrigated with noxythiolin (2.5%) before implantation. Later in the same study, gentamicin solution (80 mg/l) was substituted for noxythiolin, and this was used to soak the wound packs as well as to irrigate the shunt system before implantation. This resulted in a statistically significant fall in the incidence of shunt infection compared to when noxythiolin was used, and compared to the use of adhesive drapes without wound packs. No systemic antibiotics were administered. The incidence of shunt infection in 318 operations where gentamicin solution was used was 0.94%.

* Geistlich and Sons Ltd, Newton Bank, Long Lane, Chester CH2 3QZ.

Fitzgerald and Connelly (1984) used a similar system, except that all patients in their study also received intramuscular cloxacillin to protect specifically against wound infection. After shaving in the operating theatre by the surgeon, a methodical skin preparation was carried out using Phisomed (hexachlorophane) followed by aqueous povidone-iodine, then aqueous chlorhexidine to the incision sites. The surgeon then rescrubbed. Cloth wound drapes soaked in aqueous chlorhexidine were used and extra ones similarly treated were applied to protect the wound edges. The shunt was flushed with gentamicin and soaked in this before implantation. A 'no-touch' technique was used. In 82 consecutive operations there were 2 shunt infections (2.4%) both due to coagulase-negative staphylococci. This compares to a rate of approximately 7% before this study was begun. Unfortunately, the study was not randomized and could perhaps be criticized on the grounds that it was sequential and had no control group. However, like Tabara and Forrest (1982) the authors used gentamicin to irrigate the shunt and an antibacterial agent to soak the drapes at the wound edges. One or both of these measures, along with sound surgical technique, might have been responsible for the improvements in infection rate.

6.6 PROPHYLACTIC ANTIBIOTICS

The use of systemic prophylactic antibiotics appears to be an obvious method of reducing the incidence of shunt infection, especially following its proven beneficial effect in other forms of surgery. However, this is yet another instance of the need to consider cerebrospinal fluid shunt surgery separately from other operative procedures. When considering the effectiveness of antibiotic prophylaxis it is also essential to evaluate true shunt colonization as defined in Chapter 2 separately from external shunt infections. When associated with shunt surgery, rather than as a result of later erosion, these latter are really wound infections involving a foreign body and the principles of their prevention are different. This is only one reason why most studies of the role of antibiotic prophylaxis in this field are incapable of reliable interpretation, and therefore are often wrongly interpreted, as the known effect on wound infection is not distinguished from any effect on true shunt infection rate. Certainly the use of antibiotics in this way is controversial.

Before the well-defined period of risk associated with shunt surgery was appreciated, it was assumed that the implanted shunt presented a continuing risk of infection and this led Holt (1970) to consider the long-term administration of fusidic acid. However, in most cases the use of prophylactic antibiotics has been confined to the operative period. As most shunt infections are caused by staphylococci, those workers who have used antibiotics have usually used antistaphylococcal ones, and that most often used in American reports is methicillin, though Venes (1976) recommended oxacillin.

6.7   STUDIES USING SYSTEMIC ANTIBIOTICS

Some of the reports of 'trials' of the use of prophylactic antibiotics suffer from the fact that the control group is studied before the prophylaxis group. In other words they are studied sequentially and often retrospectively. McCullough *et al.* (1980) studied 257 patients in this way. Before the end of 1974, antibiotics were not used and the infection rate was 8% of operations. From 1975 to 1978 all patients in the study were given methicillin, either intramuscularly or intravenously, starting immediately preoperatively and continuing for 36 hours postoperatively. During this second period the operative infection rate was 2.6%. Similarly, Ajir, Levin and Duff (1981) studied two groups of patients sequentially, giving the second group a single preoperative intravenous dose of methicillin. In those patients undergoing primary shunt insertions, of 73 who received no prophylaxis, 4 (5.5%) became infected, whereas 3 of the next 34 who received antibiotics developed shunt infections. The difference is not statistically significant, though the authors claim a statistically significant difference between the infection rates for revisions, there being none in the prophylaxis group.

In a retrospective study over 25 years and involving 840 patients, George, Leibrock and Epstein (1979) found that the uncontrolled use of antibiotics, chiefly methicillin, had no effect on the infection rate, and that infections in the prophylaxis group were usually due to organisms which were susceptible to the drug used, an observation made by others.

Ivan, Choo and Ventureyra (1980) also carried out a sequential study over four years involving 125 patients. Routine use of either cloxacillin or a cephalosporin for prophylaxis was begun towards the end of the study and this was apparently followed by a fall in the infection rate. However, close analysis of the figures strongly suggests that the annual number of infections was already falling before the start of antibiotic prophylaxis. The authors state that there was a more standardized approach at about this time, and that 'neither operative technique nor the use of prophylactic antibiotics was uniform until 1976 (half-way through the study), when the shunt operation was done by fewer surgeons resulting in a decline of shunt infections'. George, Leibrock and Epstein (1979) also noted that infections became less frequent during their study. This is, as Haines (1980) points out in his valuable critical review, one of the major disadvantages of a sequential study.

Almost inevitably improvements are made in operative technique or equipment, and it is virtually impossible for those involved at all levels, to retain throughout the study the level of knowledge and experience which pertains at its beginning. This and the heightening of interest and awareness merely because the study is taking place, is the Hawthorn Effect (Entwistle and Nisbet, 1972).

Yu and Patterson (1973) also carried out a retrospective review of 160 cases, one-third of whom received an antistaphylococcal drug intravenously. This was started within the first day or two postoperatively and continued for five days.

Various drugs were used and the numbers for each drug were small. Moreover, there was no attempt at randomization or control, and the decision of whether or not to use prophylaxis was made by the individual surgeon using criteria which are not stated. The authors report a difference in infection rate between those not receiving prophylaxis (19%) and those who did (2%). This study would appear at first sight to support the use of antibiotics but because of the problems referred to, it is impossible to evaluate.

In another uncontrolled study in which methicillin and dicloxacillin were used, Ignelzi and Kirsch (1975) failed to show a significant fall in infection rate over two years. Pui, Lawrence and Vanderzwagg (1981), using ampicillin, oxacillin and gentamicin, studied 133 cases and found no beneficial effect, though the study was retrospective and was not randomized.

Malis (1979) studied 1732 cases involving neurosurgical procedures, including 128 shunt operations. He used intramuscular tobramycin and intravenous vancomycin immediately preoperatively, and used an irrigating fluid containing streptomycin. He claims to have had no infections at all in any of the 1732 cases, and therefore by implication in the 128 shunt cases. However, this study was prompted by failure of an earlier study using prophylactic clindamycin, during which there was an outbreak of infection. Again therefore, the study was in one sense a sequential one. More important perhaps is the definition and follow-up of wound infection, which led to exclusion of an unknown number of infections which were deemed to be due to postoperative aspiration of fluid collections in the wound. The study is much more concerned with the prevention of infection in general neurosurgery than with shunt infections and one wonders about the criteria used for diagnosis of shunt infection in this study.

A prospective randomized study was carried out by Bayston (1975), in which 20 patients received gentamicin, and 34 received cloxacillin, both given intravenously on induction of anaesthesia. A further dose was administered six hours after the first. A control group of 78 patients received no antibiotic prophylaxis. Blood cultures were taken within one hour of the operation, and beta-lactamase was added to those which were from patients receiving cloxacillin.

None of the blood cultures from those patients receiving gentamicin grew organisms, whereas 24% of the cloxacillin group and 27% of the controls, respectively were positive. The operative incisions were sampled before closure using a velvet pad impression technique (Holt) and 60%, 63% and 51% of the wounds in the gentamicin, cloxacillin and control groups respectively grew organisms. These were usually staphylococci and were usually fully susceptible *in vitro* to the drugs used.

During the operation, a small piece of tissue was removed and tested for antibiotic activity; all of those from the antibiotic groups were positive. There was, therefore, a paradoxical situation of demonstrable achievement of antibacterial tissue levels coinciding with presence of viable, susceptible contaminating organisms in the incisions. This can of course be explained by the failure of culture techniques to demonstrate bacteria already killed or irreversibly damaged by the antibiotic, along with their constant replacement by viable organisms entering the wounds from the skin. However, as we have previously shown (Bayston and Lari, 1974) that shunt infections usually result from skin organisms entering the surgical wound at operation, we felt this finding to be important.

The absence of organisms in blood cultures from the gentamicin group was probably due to the effect of antibiotics in the blood. No attempt was made to inactivate the gentamicin, whereas the cloxacillin was neutralized. The blood culture results are therefore not very helpful, and we have shown that the organisms usually involved in the apparent postoperative bacteraemia following shunt surgery are not those which subsequently colonize the shunts (Bayston and Lari, 1974). It is not surprising, therefore, that the authors found no significant difference between the three groups in terms of either wound infection or true shunt infection. Unfortunately for the study, the numbers of each were very small and this detracted from the value of the analysis.

Haines and Taylor (1982) used methicillin intravenously or intramuscularly in a double-blind randomized controlled trial involving 74 children. From a total of 7 infections (9.5%), 5 (12.8%) occurred in the placebo group and 2 (5.7%) in the methicillin group. All patients had ventriculoperitoneal shunts and the authors also report a number of malfunctions which they do not ascribe to infection. There is a different distribution of malfunctions in terms of time between the two groups, the placebo group having a statistically significant rise in incidence between one and four and a half months. These authors suggest that methicillin might prevent such delayed malfunction. The relationship between malfunction and infection in ventriculoperitoneal shunts has been discussed (see Chapter 2). While malfunction due to infection usually appears within three months of operation, the use of serological surveillance (see Chapter 4) might have detected infection in some of these delayed malfunctioning shunts, thus explaining the apparent protective effect of methicillin as merely delaying presentation. However, the incidence of malfunction overall is not significantly different in either group, and even if some were due to infection the authors' conclusion that prophylactic methicillin has no protective effect against shunt infection would not be invalidated.

A different antibiotic, vancomycin, was used by Odio *et al.* (1984) in a randomized double-blind controlled trial involving 37 cases. The drug was administered intravenously one hour before operation, with another dose six hours later. All infections were due to staphylococci and all were, of course, susceptible to the drug *in vitro*. There was no significant difference in infection rates between the vancomycin group (17%) and the placebo group (23%). Moreover, 7 patients (35%) had an adverse reaction to the drug and the trial had to be terminated early.

6.8 STUDIES USING INTRAVENTRICULAR ANTIBIOTICS

One probable reason for the failure of intravenous drugs to prevent shunt infection is the very low levels achieved in the cerebrospinal fluid (McCullough *et al.*, 1980). This especially explains the results of Odio *et al.*

Salmon (1972) used methicillin both intravenously and intraventricularly preoperatively, in 32 patients. His infection rate, previously 19% dropped to 3% (one case). While recognizing the problems associated with sequential studies, the author considered these results to be encouraging. Welch (1977), in a sequential study, compared the infection rate in 186 cases during a period when prophylactic antibiotics were not routinely used with a consecutive group of 197 cases who all received antibiotics.

Those in the second group received a variety of antibiotics intravenously, but 150 received an intraventricular antibiotic, almost all gentamicin, in addition. The rate of true shunt infection in the first period was 4.3% (8 cases) 5 of these having received systemic antibiotics. During the second group, in which all patients received systemic antibiotics, the rate was 1%. This consisted of 2 cases in the group not receiving intraventricular drugs, and none amongst those who did.

Unfortunately, the numbers in both groups are small. The author also points out that there were other possible factors contributory to the lower incidence, such as the soaking of the shunts in a solution of polymyxin B before implantation, improvements to the operating suite and alterations to the surgical technique, including introduction of a 'no-touch' method. A further interesting aspect of this paper is the account of untoward events associated with the use of intraventricular gentamicin. One patient who received both intravenous and intraventricular gentamicin developed severe high-tone hearing loss. Two others also developed hearing loss but in one this predated the operation and in the other no preoperative audiogram was available. Most patients received 5 mg of gentamicin intraventricularly, but 1 patient who received 10 mg experienced distortion of hearing ten days later, which subsided leaving a conductive deficit. Seizures occurred in 2 patients. Again, 1 received 10 mg and the second, while receiving 5 mg had slit ventricles and a low cerebrospinal fluid volume of distribution. These experiences must serve as a caveat for anyone using intraventricular aminoglycosides for prophylaxis, and overdosage should apparently be avoided for the same reasons as when the drugs are used systemically.

A prospective randomized trial was carried out by Lambert, McKinnon and Vaishnav (1984). These workers compared three groups of patients, all of whom had a standard thorough skin preparation preoperatively using povidone-iodine. Twenty patients who received no antibiotics formed the control group, and a further 24 had their incisions irrigated throughout the operation with aqueous povidone-iodine as well as having their shunts 'cleaned' externally with this solution before implantation. The third group received a single intravenous dose of gentamicin preoperatively and a single dose of the same drug at the conclusion of surgery, injected above the level of revision, that is intraventricularly or into the proximal shunt as appropriate. Five milligrams were usually used but 10 mg were injected if the ventricles were very dilated. The overall infection rate was 13.2%. There were 4 infections in the control group (20%) and 4 in the povidone-iodine group (17%) but only 1 in the gentamicin group. This infection was due to an alpha-haemolytic streptococcus which was resistant to gentamicin, whereas the other infections were due to coagulase-negative staphylococci.

If this resistant organism is excluded from the analysis, the difference in infection rate between the gentamicin group and the control group is statistically significant according to the tests used by the authors, but again the numbers are small. These workers prospectively excluded cases from the trial where gentamicin-resistant strains were found on the skin before operation. They also used serological surveillance (Bayston 1975, see Chapter 4) to increase the reliability of their detection of shunt infection.

From most of these studies, support for an opinion either for or against the use of prophylactic antibiotics can be derived, as Haines (1980) states in his review. Ideally, a large randomized double-blind study should be undertaken in order to avoid the methodological pitfalls of most earlier studies, and to provide enough patients for an unequivocal statistical evaluation to be made. Because of its very nature, this is a daunting task which is unlikely to be undertaken. One must also consider that, if statistics and very large numbers are necessary to show a beneficial effect of prophylactic antibiotics in this field, then whatever the outcome the effect is unlikely to be great.

The question would therefore arise of the ultimate worth in terms of case management. This is particularly so if one is to take account of possible undesirable and toxic effects.

However, there is some suggestion from previous studies that, if antibiotic prophylaxis is to be used, the drugs must be given intraventricularly to have an effect on true shunt infection. This is also in accordance with what we know about the aetiology of shunt infection. The choice of drug should be dictated by its toxicity, its antibacterial spectrum and its bactericidal effect.

Welch's (1977) work suggests that aminoglycosides are not as safe as was once thought when given intraventricularly. They are also very poorly active against propionibacteria, which are being isolated with increasing frequency from infected shunts. Methicillin might be effective, as Salmon suggests, but there are doubts about its bactericidal effect in such circumstances.

Vancomycin sometimes leads to thrombophlebitis or histamine-like reactions when administered by the intravenous route (Odio *et al.*, 1984) but appears to be both safe and effective when given intraventricularly (Visconti and Peters, 1979; Raoult *et al.*, 1981; Sutherland *et al.*, 1981; Young, Ratner and Clarridge, 1981; Bayston *et al.*, 1984; Andrew and Waters, 1986; Swayne, Rampling and Newsom, 1987; Bayston, Hart and Barnicoat, 1987). Also there is laboratory evidence that it prevents bacterial adhesion even in low doses (Bernard, Francioli and Glauser, 1981). At the time of writing, a randomized trial of intraventricular vancomycin in shunt surgery is under way under the auspices of the United Kingdom Shunt Discussion Group, involving 800 patients. Vancomycin is active against all strains of staphylococci, and most other Gram-positive organisms likely to be found in shunts, such as coryneforms (including the 'JK' group), propionibacteria and most enterococci. Teicoplanin, a related antibiotic may also be effective but further work is needed on this drug.

From the foregoing, certain factors appear to be noteworthy. A method of preventing skin organisms from entering the immediate operative area of the incision, such as those used by Tabara and Forrest (1982) and Fitzgerald and Connelly (1984), accords with a known risk factor and is more likely to be effective than systemic antibiotics. The method employed by Lambert, McKinnon and Vaishnav (1984), of irrigating the incisions during the operation with povidone-iodine, may have a similar effect. The other factor which is likely to be important is the use of an appropriate antibiotic in such a way that it is in contact with any bacteria which circumvent the antimicrobial skin barriers – and some certainly will – and gain entry to the shunt lumen. Either the drug should be introduced directly into the cerebral ventricles during the operation, or the shunt should be irrigated and soaked in it before implantation. Intraventricular instillation of gentamicin as practised by Welch (1977) and Lambert, McKinnon and Vaishnav (1984), or possibly methicillin (Salmon, 1972) or preferably vancomycin, or the use of gentamicin to irrigate the shunt system (Tabara and Forrest 1982; Fitzgerald and Connelly, 1984; Lambert, McKinnon and Vaishnav, 1984) appear likely to enhance protection.

Such methods are likely to be ineffective, however, if they are not accompanied by meticulous aseptic technique, the introduction, for example, of a 'no-touch' method, and a high level of surgical expertise. In addition, part of the training of surgeons involved in this field should be devoted to bringing about a full understanding of the nature of the very special problems of implant infections. Those surgeons who believe that shunt insertion or revision is 'just another operation' are likely to encounter considerable problems with shunt infections.

6.9   PROPHYLAXIS FOR DENTAL SURGERY

Another time when antibiotic prophylaxis is often prescribed is when a shunted patient is about to undergo dental treatment. There is little published information on the risk at such a time to the shunt, but the author has sought, and failed to find, any connection between dental treatment and any of his infections. Penicillin or amoxycillin is often used in the UK as in those at risk of endocarditis, but these are most unlikely to have any effect on the usual infecting organisms in shunts in any case, so effective dental prophylaxis for shunted patients is probably not practised, and is almost certainly not required.

6.10   ANTIBACTERIAL CATHETERS

Another, as yet experimental, method of possible prophylaxis is that of impregnation of the whole shunt material with antimicrobial substances so that bacteria coming into contact with it will be killed. Various methods of doing this have been described (Bayston and

Milner, 1981) and it has been shown that the technique can be manipulated to achieve a period of continuing antibacterial activity of up to three years after constant perfusion of the impregnated catheters in the laboratory. Of course, in the case of cerebrospinal fluid shunts, the period of risk is much shorter (see Chapter 2) and the required few days' activity can easily be attained. This work is being pursued with a view to using antibacterial shunts in, for example, high-risk patients or where there is an abnormally high incidence of shunt infection.

6.11 RECOMMENDATIONS FOR CURRENT PRACTICE

1. Shave in anaesthetic room or preferably use depilatory cream on ward;
2. Thorough skin preparation with hexachlorophane detergent (e.g. Phisomed) or possibly iodophore, (e.g. povidone-iodine) followed by alcoholic chlorhexidine. As there is a slight risk of neurotoxicity if chlorhexidine comes into contact with brain tissue, it is essential to avoid contamination of the ventricular catheter with the antiseptic.
3. Drapes in the vicinity of the incisions should either be impervious or be soaked in aqueous chlorhexidine;
4. Wound edge packs, soaked in aqueous chlorhexidine, should be used and properly applied. As there is a slight risk of neurotoxicity if chlorhexidine comes into contact with brain tissue, it is essential to avoid contamination of the ventricular catheter with the antiseptic.
5. One intraventricular dose of either gentamicin (up to 5 mg) or vancomycin (10–20 mg) should be given peroperatively;
6. The shunt for implantation should be irrigated and immersed in a solution of the same agent before use;
7. No further antibiotics should be given unless otherwise indicated, for example by an increased risk of wound infection;
8. Excellent surgical technique and an appreciation of the problems of shunt surgery should be developed and encouraged in others.

REFERENCES

Acocella, G., Bonollo, L., Mainardi, M. *et al.* (1977) Serum and urine concentrations of rifampicin administered by intravenous infusion in man. (Arzneim, Forsch.) *Drug Research*, **27** (1), 1221–6.

Ajir, F., Levin, A. B. and Duff, T. A. (1981) Effect of prophylactic methicillin on cerebrospinal fluid shunt infections in children. *Neurosurgery*, **9** (1), 6–8.

Allen, K. D. and Green, H. T. (1986) Infections due to a 'Group JK' Coryneforms. *J. Infect.*, **13**, 41–4.

Anderson, F. M. (1959) Ventriculo-auriculostomy in treatment of hydrocephalus. *J. Neurosurg.*, **16**, 551–7.

Anderson, H. C. and McCarty, M. (1950) Determination of C-reactive protein in blood as a measure of activity of disease process in acute rheumatic fever. *Am. J. Med.*, **8**, 445–55.

Andrew, J. H. and Waters, M. J. (1986) Hydrocephalus shunt infections and their treatment. *J. Antimicrob. Chemother.*, **18**, 145–6.

Anker, N. and Bang, F. D. C. (1981) Longterm intravenous rifampicin treatment. Advantages and disadvantages. *Sur. J. Respir. Dis.*, **62**, 84–6.

Archer, G. L., Tenenbaum, M. J. and Haywood, H. B. (1978) Rifampicin therapy of *Staphylococcus epidermidis*. *JAMA*, **240**, (8), 751–3.

Baehr, G. and Hande, H. (1920) Glomerulonephritis as a complication of sub-acute streptococcal endocarditis. *JAMA*, **75**, 789–90.

Baird-Parker, A. C. (1963) A classification of micrococci and staphylococci based on physiological and biochemical tests. *J. Gen. Microbiol.*, **30**, 409–27.

Baird-Parker, A. C. (1965) Classification of staphylococci and micrococci from world-wide sources. *J. Gen. Microbiol.* **38**, 363–87.

Bassett, D. C., Dickson, J. A. and Hunt, G. H. (1973) Infection of Holter valve by Pseudomonas-contaminated chlorexidine. *Lancet*, **i**, 1263–4.

Bayston, R. (1971) Serological indications of *Staphylococcus albus* infection in children with colonised shunts. *Dev. Med. Child. Neurol.* (Suppl.) **25**, 135–6.

Bayston, R. (1972) Serological investigation in children with colonised Spitz–Holter valves. *J. Clin. Pathol.*, **25**, 718–20.

Bayston, R. (1975) Antibiotic prophylaxis in shunt surgery. *Dev. Med. Neurol.* (Suppl. 17) **35** 99–103.

Bayston, R. (1975) Serological surveillance of children with CSF shunting devices. *Dev. Med. Child. Neurol.* (Suppl. 17) **35**, 104–10.

Bayston, R. (1977) Studies on bacterial colonisation of cerebrospinal fluid shunting devices for the control and treatment of hydrocephalus. *M. Med. Sci. Thesis*, Univ. Sheffield.

Bayston, R. (1979) Serum C-reactive protein test in diagnosis of septic complications of cerebrospinal fluid shunts for hydrocephalus. *Arch. Dis. Child.*, **54** (7), 545–7.

Bayston, R. (1984) A model of catheter colonisation and its relationship to clinical catheter infections. *J. Infect.*, **9**, 271–6.

Bayston, R. (1987) Intraventricular vancomycin for treatment of shunt-associated ventriculitis. *J. Antimicrob. Chemother.*, **20**, 283.

Bayston, R., Barnicoat, M., Cudmore, R. E. *et al.* (1984) The use of intraventricular vancomycin in shunt-associated ventriculitis. *Z. Kinderchir.* (Suppl. 39) **II**, 111–3.

Bayston, R., Hart, C. A. and Barnicoat, M. (1987) Intraventricular vancomycin in the treatment of ventriculitis associated with cerebrospinal fluid shunting and drainage. *J. Neurol. Neurosurg. Psychiatr.*, **50**, 1419–23.

Bayston, R. and Higgins, J. (1986) Biochemical and cultural characteristics of 'JK' coryneforms. *J. Clin. Pathol.*, **39**, 654–60.

Bayston, R. and Lari, J. (1974) A study of the sources of infection in colonised shunts. *Dev. Med. Child. Neurol.* (Suppl.) **32**, 16–22.

Bayston, R., Leung, T. S., Wilkins, B. M. and Hodges, B. (1983) Bacteriological examination of removed cerebrospinal fluid shunts. *J. Clin. Pathol.*, **36** (9), 987–90.

Bayston, R. and Milner, R. D. G. (1981) Antimicrobial activity of silicone rubber used in hydrocephalus shunts, after impregnation with antimicrobial substances. *J. Clin. Pathol.*, **34**, 1057–62.

Bayston, R. and Penny, S. R. (1972) Excessive production of mucoid substance by Staphylococcus SIIA: A possible factor in colonisation of Holter shunts. *Dev. Med. Child. Neurol.* (Suppl. 14) **27**, 25–8.

Bayston, R. and Rickwood, A. M. K. (1981) Factors involved in the antibiotic treatment of cerebrospinal fluid shunt infections. *Z. Kinderchir.*, **34** (4), 339–45.

Bayston, R. and Spitz, L. (1977) Infective and cystic causes of malfunction of ventriculoperitoneal shunts for hydrocephalus. *Z. Kinderchir.*, **22** (4), 419–24.

Bayston, R. and Spitz, L. (1978) The role of retrograde movement of bacteria in ventriculoatrial shunt colonisation. *Z. Kinderchir.*, **25**, 352–6.

Bayston, R. and Swinden, J. (1979) The aetiology and prevention of shunt nephritis. *Z. Kinderchir.*, **28** (4), 377–84.

Bayston, R. and Swinden, J. (1981) Effects of test conditions on the susceptibility of staphylococci *in vitro* to cephradine, cephaloridine, cephalexin and cefuroxime. *J. Clin. Pathol.*, **34**, 203–7.

Becker, D. P. and Nulsen, F. E. (1967) Control of hydrocephalus by valve-regulated venous shunt: avoidance of complications in prolonged shunt maintenance. *J. Neurosurg.*, **28**, 215–26.

Beeler, B. A., Crowder, J. G., Smith, J. W. and White, A. (1976) *Propionibacterium acnes*: pathogen in central nervous system shunt infection. Report of three cases including immune complex glomerulonephritis. *Am. J. Med.*, **61** (6), 935–8.

Bergey's Manual of Determinative Bacteriology (1974) 8th edn, Williams & Wilkins, Baltimore.

Bernard, J. P., Francioli, P. and Glauser, M. P. (1981) Vancomycin prophylaxis of experimental *Streptococcus sanguis*. *J. Clin. Invest.*, **68** (4), 1113–16.

Bhagwati, S. N. (1971) Ventriculoatrial shunt in tuberculous meningitis with hydrocephalus. *J. Neurosurg.*, **35**, 309–13.

Birzis, L., Carter, C. H. and Maren, T. H. (1958) Effect of acetazolamide on CSF pressure and electrolytes in hydrocephalus. *Neurology (Minneap.)*, **8** (7), 522–8.

Black, J. A., Challacombe, D. N. and Ockenden, B. G. (1965) Nephrotic syndrome associated with bacteraemia after shunt operations for hydrocephalus. *Lancet*, **ii**, 921–4.

Black, W. A., Bannerman, C. M. and Black, D. A. (1974) Carriage of potentially pathogenic bacteria in the hair. *Br. J. Surg.*, **61**, 735–8.

Blackwell, C. C. and Law, J. A. (1981) Typing of non-serogroupable *Neisseria meningitidis* by means of sensitivity to R-type pyocines of *Pseudomonas aeruginosa*. *J. Infect.*, **3**, 370–8.

Blackwell, C. C., Young, H. and Anderson, I. (1979) Sensitivity of *Neisseria gonorrhoeae* to partially purified R-type pyocines and a possible approach to epidemiological typing. *J. Med. Microbiol.*, **12** (3), 321–35.

Blazé, J. B., Forrest, D. M. and Tsingoglou, S. (1971) Atriotomy using the Holter shunt in hydrocephalus. *Dev. Med. Child. Neurol.*, (Suppl. 13) **25**, 27–32.

Blowers, R., Mason, G. A., Wallace, K. R. and Walton, M. (1955) Control of wound infection in a thoracic surgery unit. *Lancet*, **ii**, 786–94.

Bolton, W. K., Sande, M. A., Normansell, D. E. *et al.* (1975) Ventriculojugular shunt nephritis with *Corynebacterium bovis*. Successful therapy with antibiotics. *Am. J. Med.*, **59** (3), 417–23.

Borges, L. F. (1982) Cerebrospinal fluid shunts interfere with host defences. *Neurosurgery*, **10** (1), 55–60.

Boughton, W. H. and Atkin, J. F. (1980) Ventricular peritoneal shunt infection caused by a member of the rhodochrous complex. *J. Clin. Microbiol.*, **II** (5), 533–4.

Boulton-Jones, J. M., Sissons, J. G. P., Evans, D. J. and Peters, D. K. (1974) Renal lesions of subacute infective endocarditis. *Br. Med. J.*, **2**, 11–14.

Brook, I., Controni, G., Rodriguez, W. J. and Martin, W. J. (1980) Anaerobic bacteraemia in children. *Am. J. Dis. Child.*, **134**, 1052–6.

Brook, I., Johnson, N., Overturf, G. and Wilkins, J. (1977) Mixed bacterial meningitis: a complication of ventriculo- and lumbo-peritoneal shunts. *J. Neurosurg.*, **47**, 961–4.

Bruce, A. M., Lorber, J., Shedden, W. I. H. and Zachary, R. B. (1963) Persistent bacteraemia following ventriculocaval shunt operations for hydrocephalus in infants. *Dev. Med. Child. Neurol.*, **5**, 461–70.

Brumfitt, W. and Pursell, R. (1972) Double-blind trial to compare ampicillin, cephalexin, co-trimoxazole and trimethoprim in treatment of urinary infection. *Br. Med. J.*, **2**, 673–6.

Bunim, J. J., Kutner, A. G., Baldwin, J. S. and McEwen, C. (1952) Cortisone and Corticotropin in rheumatic fever and juvenile rheumatoid arthritis. *JAMA*, **150**, 1273–8.

Burdon, K. L., Davis, J. S. and Wende, R. D. (1967) Experimental infection of mice with *Bacillus cereus*. Studies of pathogenesis and pathologic changes. *J. Infect. Dis.*, **117**, 307–16.

Callaghan, R. P., Cohen, S. J. and Stewart, G. T. (1961) Septicaemia due to colonisation of Spitz–Holter valves by Staphylococcus. *Br. Med. J.*, **1**, 860–3.

Caron, C., Luneau, C., Gervais, M. H. *et al.* (1979) La glomerulonephrite de shunt: manifestations cliniques et histopathologiques. *Can. Med. Assoc. J.*, **120** (5), 557–61.

Carrington, K. W. (1959) Ventriculovenous shunt using the Holter valve as a treatment of hydrocephalus. *J. Michigan Med. Soc.*, **58**, 373–6.

Castro-Gago, M., Sanguinedo, P., Garcia, C. *et al.* (1982) Valor de la proteina C-reactiva (PCR) en el diagnostico de las complicaciones infecciosas de los 'shunts' en nos niños hidrocefalos. *An. Esp. Pediatr.*, **16** (1), 47–52.

Charnley, J. and Eftekhar, N. (1969) Postoperative infection in total prosthetic replacement arthroplasty of the hip joint, with special reference to the bacterial content of the air of the operating room. *Br. J. Surg.*, **56** (9), 641–9.

Chester, D. C., Penny, S. R. and Emery, J. L. (1971) Fat-containing macrophages in the cerebrospinal fluid of children with hydrocephalus. *Dev. Med. Child. Neurol.*, (Suppl. 13) **25**, 33–8.

Chonmaitree, T., Congeni, B. L., Munoz, J. *et al.* (1984) Twice daily ceftriaxone therapy for serious bacterial infections in children. *J. Antimicrob. Chemother.*, **13**, 511–6.

Christensen, G. D., Simpson, W. A., Bisno, A. L. and Beachey, F. H. (1982) Adherence of slime-producing strains of *Staphylococcus epidermidis* to smooth surfaces. *Infect. Immunol.*, **37** (1), 318–26.

Cohen, S. J. and Callaghan, R. P. (1961) Septicaemia due to colonisation of Spitz–Holter valves by Staphylococcus. *Br. Med. J.*, **i**, 860–3.

Cohle, S. D., Hind, D. and Yawn, D. H. (1981) *Propionibacterium acnes* infection following subdural tap. *Am. J. Clin. Pathol.*, **75** (3), 430–1.

Corrall, C. J., Pepple, J. M., Moxon, E. R. and Hughes, W. T. (1981) C-reactive protein in spinal fluid of children with meningitis. *J. Pediatr.*, **99** (3), 365–7.

Cox, R., Sockwell, G. and Landers, B. (1959) *Bacillus cereus* septicaemia: report of a case and review of the literature. *N. Engl. J. Med.*, **261**, 894–6.

Crockson, R. A., Payne, C. J., Ratcliffe, A. P. and Soothill, J. F. (1966) Time sequence of acute phase reactive proteins following surgical trauma. *Clin. Chim. Acta*, **14**, 435–41.

Darrell, J. H., Garrod, L. P. and Waterworth, P. M. (1968) Trimethoprim: Laboratory and clinical studies. *J. Clin. Pathol.*, **21**, 202–9.

Del Rio, M., McCracken, G. H., Nelson, J. D. *et al.* (1982) Pharmacokinetics and cerebrospinal fluid bactericidal activity of ceftriaxone in the treatment of pediatric patients with bacterial meningitis. *Antimicrob. Agents Chemother.*, **22** (6), 622–7.

Denoya, C. D., Trevisan, A. R. and Zorzopulos, J. (1986) Adherence of multiresistant strains of *Klebsiella pneumoniae* to cerebrospinal fluid shunts: correlation with plasmid content. *J. Med. Microbiol.*, **21**, 225–31.

Drachter, A. (1925) Über neue operative Weye zur Druckenlastung bei angeborenem Hydrocephalus (Ureter-Dura-Anastomose). *Zentralbl. P. Chirurg. Leipz.*, **27**, 76.

Du Boulay, G. H. (1966) Pulsatile movements in the CSF pathways. *Br. J. Radiol.*, **39**, 255–62.

Emery, J. L. and Hilton, H. B. (1961) Lung and heart complications of the treatment of hydrocephalus by ventriculo-auriculostomy. *Surgery*, **50**, 309–14.

Entwistle, N. J. and Nisbet, J. D. (1972) *Educational Research in Action*, Univ. London Press, London.

Epstein, F., Hockwald, G. and Ransohoff, J. (1973) Neonatal hydrocephalus treated by compressive head wrapping. *Lancet*, **i**, 634.

Erdohazi, M., Eckstein, H. B. and Crome, L. (1966) Pulmonary embolisation as a complication of ventriculo–atrial shunts inserted for hydrocephalus. *Dev. Med. Child. Neurol.*, (Suppl. 11) **8**, 36–44.

Everett, E. D., Eickhoff, T. C. and Simon, R. G. (1976) Cerebrospinal fluid shunt infections with anaerobic diphtheroids (propionibacterium species) *J. Neurosurg.*, **44**, 580–4.

Ezer, G. and Soothill, J. F. (1974) Intracellular bactericidal effects of rifampicin in both normal and chronic granulomatous disease polymorphs. *Arch. Dis. Child.*, **49**, 463–6.

Fahey, J. L. and McKelvey, E. M. (1965) Quantitative determination of serum immunoglobulins in antibody-agar plates. *J. Immunol.*, **94**, 84–90.

Feldman, W. E. (1976) *Bacteroides fragilis* ventriculitis and meningitis. Report of two cases. *Am. J. Dis. Child.*, **130** (8), 880–3.

Ferguson, A. H. (1898) Intraperitoneal diversion of the cerebrospinal fluid in cases of hydrocephalus. *N. Y. Med. J.*, **67**, 902–1008.

Fischer, C. L., Gill, C., Forrester, M. G. and Nakamura, R. (1976) Quantitation of 'acute phase proteins' postoperatively. Value in detection and monitoring of complications. *Am. J. Clin. Pathol.*, **66**, 840–6.

Fischer, E. G. and Shillito, J. (1969) Large abdominal cysts: a complication of peritoneal shunts. Report of three cases. *J. Neurosurg.*, **31**, 441–4.

Fischer, E. G., Shillito, J. and Schuster, S. (1972) Ventriculo–direct atrial shunts. A clinical evaluation. *J. Neurosurg.*, **36**, 438–40.

Fishman, R. A. (1966) Blood–brain and CSF barriers to penicillin and related organic acids. *Arch. Neurol.*, **15**, 113–24.

Fitzgerald, R. and Connelly, B. (1984) An operative technique to reduce valve colonisation. *Z. Kinderchir.*, **39**, (Suppl. II) 107–9.

Fokes, E. C. (1970) Occult infections of ventriculo–atrial shunts. *J. Neurosurg.*, **33**, 517–23.

Forrest, D. M. and Cooper, D. G. W. (1968) Complications of ventriculoatrial shunts. A review of 455 cases. *J. Neurosurg.*, **29**, 506–12.

Futrakul, P., Suprapathana, L. and Campbell, R. A. (1970) Review of shunt nephritis. *J. Med. Assoc. Thai.*, **53** (4), 265–72.

Gardner, A. D. (1948) Rapid disinfection of clean unwashed skin. *Lancet*, **ii**, 760–3.

Gardner, A. D. and Seddon, H. J. (1946) Rapid chemical disinfection of clean unwashed skin. *Lancet*, **i**, 583–6.

Garrod, L. P. (1937) The susceptibility of different bacteria to destruction in the stomach. *J. Pathol. Bacteriol.*, **45**, 473–4.

George, R., Leibrock, L. and Epstein, M. (1979) Longterm analysis of cerebrospinal fluid shunt infections. A 25-year experience. *J. Neurosurg.*, **51** (6), 804–11.

Gombert, M. E., Landesman, S. H., Corrado, M. L. *et al.* (1981) Vancomycin and rifampicin therapy for *Staphylococcus epidermidis* meningitis associated with CSF shunts. *J. Neurosurg.*, **55**, 633–6.

Gonzales, E. P., Crosby, R. M. and Walker, S. H. (1971) *Mycobacterium aquae* infection in a hydrocephalic child. *Pediatr.*, **48**, 974–7.

Gray, E. D., Peters, G., Verstegen, M. and Regelman, W. E. (1984) Effect of extracellular slime substance from *Staphylococcus epidermidis* on the human cellular immune response. *Lancet*, **i**, 365–7.

Green, C. E., Cameron, H. J. and Julian, G. R. (1975) Recovery of polysome function of +4-infected *Escherichia coli* after brief treatment with chloramphenicol and rifampicin. *Antimicrob. Agents Chemother.*, **7**, 549–54.

Greenwood, D. and O'Grady, F. (1972) The effect of osmolarity on the response of *Escherichia coli* and *Proteus mirabilis* to penicillins. *Br. J. Exp. Pathol.*, **53**, 457–64.

Grosfeld, J. L., Cooney, O. R., Smith, J. and Campbell, R. L. (1974) Intra-abdominal complications following ventriculoperitoneal shunt procedures. *Pediatr.*, **54**, 791–6.

Gruneberg, R. N., Emmerson, A. M. and Ridgway, G. L. (1984) Rifampicin-containing antibiotic combinations in the treatment of difficult infections. *J. Antimicrob. Chemother.*, (Suppl. C), 49–55.

Gupta, R. S. (1975) Killing and lysis of *Escherichia coli* in the presence of chloramphenicol: relation to cellular magnesium. *Antimicrob. Agents Chemother.*, **7**, 748–53.

Haines, S. J. (1980) Systemic antibiotic prophylaxis in neurological surgery. *Neurosurgery*, **6** (4), 355–61.

Haines, S. J. and Taylor, F. (1982) Prophylactic methicillin for shunt operations: effects on incidence of shunt malfunction and infection. *Child's Brain*, **9**, 10–22.

Hande, K. R., Witebsky, F. G., Brown, M. S. *et al.* (1976) Sepsis with a new species of corynebacterium. *Ann. Intern. Med.*, **85**, 423–6.

Harsh, G. R. (1954) Peritoneal shunt for hydrocephalus utilising fimbriae of the Fallopian tube for entrance to the peritoneal cavity. *J. Neurosurg.*, **II**, 284–94.

Hartmann, R., Holtje, J. and Schwarz, U. (1972) Targets of penicillin action in *Escherichia coli*. *Nature*, **235**, 426–9.

Hartwell (1913) *Ann. Surg.*, **57**, 449–84.

Harwick, H. J., Kalmanson, G. M. and Guze, L. B. (1973) *In vitro* activity of ampicillin or vancomycin combined with gentamicin or streptomycin against enterococci. *Antimicrob. Agents Chemother.*, **4**, 383–7.

Hawley, H. B. and Gump, D. W. (1973) Vancomycin therapy of bacterial meningitis. *Am. J. Dis. Child.*, **126**, 261–4.

Hayden, P. W., Foltz, E. L. and Shurtleff, D. B. (1968) Effect of an oral osmotic agent on ventricular fluid pressure of hydrocephalic children. *Pediatr.*, **41**, 955–67.

Haynes, I. S. (1913) Congenital internal hydrocephalus: its treatment by drainage of the cisterna magna into the cranial sinuses. *Ann. Surg.*, **57**, 449–84.

Heck, A. F., Hameroff, S. B. and Hornick, R. B. (1971) Chronic *Listeria monocytogenes* meningitis and normotensive hydrocephalus. *Neurology.*, **21**, 263–70.

Heile, B. (1925) Über neue operative Wege zur Druckenlastung bei borenem Hydrocephalus (Ureter-Dura-Anastomose) *Zentralbl. P. Chirurg. Leipz.*, **iii**, 2229–36.

Hieber, J. P. and Nelson, J. D. (1977) A pharmacologic evaluation of penicillin in children with purulent meningitis. *N. Engl. J. Med.*, **297**, 410–13.

Hodges, G. R., Watanabe, I., Singer, P. *et al.* (1981) Central nervous system toxicity of intraventricularly administered gentamicin in adult rabbits. *J. Infect. Dis.*, **143**, 148–55.

Holland, N. (1967) Hypocomplementemic glomerulonephritis associated with Micrococcus infection of a ventriculo–atrial shunt. *Soc. Pediatr. Res. 37th Annual Meeting*, 124.

Holt, R. J. (1966) Pad cultures on skin surfaces. *J. Appl. Bacteriol.*, **29**, 625–30.

Holt, R. (1969) The classification of staphylococci from colonised ventriculo–atrial shunts. *J. Clin. Pathol.*, **22**, 475–82.

Holt, R. J. (1970) Bacteriological studies of colonised ventriculo–atrial shunts. *Dev. Med. Child. Neurol.*, (Suppl.) **22**, 83–7.

Holt, R. (1980) The early serological detection of colonisation by *Staphylococcus epidermidis* of ventriculo–atrial shunts. *Infection*, **8** (1), 8–12.

Hufnagel, C. A., Walter, C. W. and Howard, R. W. (1948) An *in vitro* method for evaluation of detergents and germicides. *Surgery*, **23**, 753–61.

Huttenlocher, P. R. (1965) Treatment of hydrocephalus with acetazolamide: results in 15 cases. *J. Pediatr.*, **66**, 1023–30.

Ignelzi, R. J. and Kirsch, W. M. (1975) Follow-up analysis of ventriculoperitoneal and ventriculo–atrial shunts for hydrocephalus. *J. Neurosurg.*, **42** (6), 679–82.

Ivan, L. P., Choo, S. H. and Ventureyra, E. C. (1980) Complications of ventriculo–atrial and ventriculoperitoneal shunts in a new children's hospital. *Can. J. Surg.*, **23** (6), 566–8.

Ives, H. R. and Hirshfeld, J. W. (1939) The bacterial flora of clean surgical wounds. *Ann. Surg.*, **107** (4), 607–17.

Jackson, D. W., Pollock, A. V. and Tindall, D. S. (1971) The value of a plastic adhesive drape in the prevention of wound infection. A controlled trial. *Br. J. Surg.*, **58**, 340–2.

James, H. E., Walsh, J. W., Wilson, H. D. *et al.* (1980) Prospective randomised study of therapy in cerebrospinal fluid shunt infection. *Neurosurg.*, **7** (5), 459–63.

Jayne-Williams, D. J. and Skerman, T. M. (1966) Comparative studies on coryneform bacteria from milk and dairy sources. *J. Appl. Bacteriol.*, **29**, 72–92.

Jepson, O. B. (1972) Post-operative wound sepsis in general surgery. VI: The occurrence of infection with staphylococci. *Acta Chir. Scand.*, **138**, 335–41.

Johnson, W. D. and Kaye, D. (1970) Serious infections caused by diphtheroids. *Ann. NY Acad. Sci.*, **174**, 568–76.

Jordan, D. C. and Inniss, W. E. (1959) Selective inhibition of ribonucleic acid synthesis in *Staphylococcus aureus* by vancomycin. *Nature*, **184**, 1894–5.

Kaplan, K. and Weinstein, L. (1969) Diphtheroid infection of man. *Ann. Intern. Med.*, **70**, 919–29.

Kasanen, A., Toivanen, P., Sourander, L. *et al.* (1974) Trimethoprim in the treatment and long term control of urinary tract infection. *Scand. J. Infect. Dis.*, **6**, 91–6.

Katz, M. D., Rapp, R. P. and Walsh, J. W. (1980) Infection in a functioning ventriculoperitoneal shunt treated with intraventricular gentamicin. *Am. J. Hosp. Pharm.*, **37** (2), 268–71.

Kaufman, D. B. and McIntosh, H. (1971) The pathogenesis of the renal lesion in a patient with streptococcal disease, infected ventriculo–atrial shunt, cryoglobulinaemia and nephritis. *Am. J. Med.*, **50**, 262–8.

Kausch, J. (1905) Die Abteilung für Bacteriologie und experimental Therapie der deutschen Medizinischen. Ausstellung auf der Welttausstellung zu St Louis 1 ABT **xxxvi**, 593–613.

Kelly, M. C., Smith, I. D., Anstey, R. J. *et al.* (1984) Rapid identification of antibiotic-resistant corynebacteria with the API 20S system. *J. Clin. Microbiol.*, **19** (2), 245–7.

Keucher, T. R. and Mealey, J. (1979) Long term results after ventriculo–atrial and ventriculoperitoneal shunting for infantile hydrocephalus. *J. Neurosurg.*, **50** (2), 179–86.

Kindmark, C. O. (1976) Sequential changes in plasma proteins in various acute diseases. In *Plasma Protein Turnover* (ed. R. Bianchi *et al.*) Univ. Park Press, Baltimore.

Kissling, M., Bergamini, N. and Xilinas, M. (1982) Parenteral rifampicin (Rimactan iv) in tuberculous and severe non-mycobacterial infections. *Chemotherapy*, **28** (3), 229–39.

Kloos, W. E. and Schleifer, K. H. (1975) Simplified scheme for routine identification of human staphylococcus species. *J. Clin. Microbiol.*, **1** (1), 82–8.

Kourtopoulos, H. and Holm, S. (1976) Intraventricular treatment of *Serratia marcescens* meningitis with gentamicin. *Scand. J. Infect. Dis.*, **8** (1), 57–60.

Krontz, D. P. and Strausbaugh, L. J. (1980) Effect of meningitis and probenecid on the penetration of vancomycin into cerebrospinal fluid in rabbits. *Antimicrob. Agents Chemother.*, **18** (6), 882–6.

Lajat, Y., Lebatard-Sartre, R. and Guihard, D. (1975) Etude comparative des complications observées dans les dérivations ventriculo–atriales et ventriculo-péritonéales. *Neurochirurgie*, **21** (2), 147–61.

Lambert, M., McKinnon, A. E. and Vaishnav, A. (1984) Comparison of two methods of prophylaxis against CSF shunt infections. *Z. Kinderchir.*, **39**, (Suppl. II), 109–10.

Lancet Editorial (1983) How does *Brucella abortus* infect human beings. *Lancet*, **ii**, 1180–1.

Latchaw, J. P. and Hahn, J. F. (1981) Intraperitoneal pseudocyst associated with peritoneal shunt. *Neurosurg.*, **8**, 469–72.

Leffert, H. L., Batist, J. N. and Gidez, L. I. (1970) Meningitis and bacteraemia after ventriculo–atrial shunt revision: isolation of a lecithinase-producing *Bacillus cereus*. *J. Infect. Dis.*, **122** (6), 547–52.

Leggiadro, R. J., Atluru, V. L. and Katz, S. P. (1984) Meningococcal meningitis associated with cerebrospinal fluid shunts. *Pediatr. Infect. Dis.*, **3** (5), 489–90.

Lerman, S. J. (1981) *Haemophilus influenzae* infections of cerebrospinal fluid shunts. Report of two cases. *J. Neurosurg.*, **54** (2), 261–3.

Lidwell, O. M., Lowbury, E. J. L., Whyte, W. *et al.* (1982) Effect of ultraclean air in operating rooms on deep sepsis in the joint after total hip or knee replacement: a randomised study. *Br. Med. J.*, **325**, 10–14.

Lim, B. T., Avezaat, C. J. and Michel, M. F. (1980) Het voorkomen van propionibacterium acnes in bloed en liquor van neurochirurgische patienten. *Ned. Tijdschr. Geneeskd.*, **124** (17), 628–32.

Little, J. R., Rhoton, A. L. and Mellinger, J. F. (1972) Comparison of ventriculoperitoneal and ventriculo–atrial shunts for hydrocephalus in children. *Mayo Clinic. Proc.*, **47**, 396–401.

Lorber, J. (1973) The use of isosorbide in the treatment of hydrocephalus. *Dev. Med. Child. Neurol.*, (Suppl.) **27**, 87–93.

Lorber J., Rhoton, A. L. and Mellinger, J. F. (1970) Treatment of ventriculitis with gentamicin and cloxacillin in infants born with spina bifida *Arch. Dis. Child.*, **45**, 178–85.

Luthardt, T. H. (1970) Bacterial infections in ventriculo–auricular shunt systems. *Devl. Med. Child. Neurol.*, **22**, (Suppl.) 105–7.

Luthy, R., Blaser, J., Bonetti, A. *et al.* (1981) Comparative multiple-dose pharmocokinetics of cefotaxime, moxalactam, and ceftazidime. *Antimicrob. Agents Chemother.*, **20** (5), 567–75.

Macheret, H., Cruchaud, A., Junod, A. *et al.* (1974) Pneumopathie à complexes immuns au cours d'une septicémie à staphylocoque blanc: une complication in-habituelle des valves de Spitz–Holter. *Schweiz. Med. Wochenschr.*, **104**, 1771–3.

Magee, J. T., Hindmarch, J. M. and Meechan, D. F. (1983) Identification of staphylococci and micrococci. *J. Clin. Pathol.*, **35** (6), 650–6.

Males, S., Glaser, J. and Shapiro, K. (1982) Treatment of cerebrospinal fluid shunt infections with medical therapy alone. *Neurosurgery.*, **11** (6), 781–3.

Malis, L. I. (1979) Prevention of neurosurgical infection by intra-operative antibiotics. *Neurosurgery.*, **5** (3), 339–43.

Mandell, G. L. (1973) Interaction of intraleukocytic bacteria and antibiotics. *J. Clin. Invest.*, **52**, 1673–9.

Mandell, G. L. and Moorman, D. R. (1980) Treatment of experimental staphylococcal infections: Effect of rifampin alone and in combination on development of rifampin resistance. *Antimicrob. Agents Chemother.*, **17** (4), 658–62.

Maniaitis, A. and Vassilouthis, J. (1980) *Propionibacterium acnes* infection complicating craniotomy. *J. Hosp. Infect.*, **1**, 261–4.

Marples, M. J. (1965) In *Ecology of Human Skin*. C. C. Thomas, Illinois.

Marples, R. R. and Richardson, J. F. (1982) Evaluation of a micro method gallery (API Staph.) for the identification of staphylococci and micrococci. *J. Clin. Pathol.*, **35** (6), 650–6.

Marrie, T., Noble, M. A. and Costerton, J. W. (1983) Examination of the morphology of bacteria adhering to peritoneal dialysis catheters by scanning and transmission electron microscopy. *J. Clin. Microbiol.*, **18** (6), 1388–98.

Matson, D. D. (1949) New operations for treatment of communicating hydrocephalus. Report of a case secondary to generalised meningitis. *J. Neurosurg.*, **6**, 238–47.

McCarthy, M. F. and Wenzel, R. P. (1977) Postoperative spinal fluid infections after neurosurgical shunting procedures. *Pediatrics*, **59** (5), 793.

McCullough, D. C., Kane, J. G., Presper, J. H. and Wells, M. (1980) Antibiotic prophylaxis in ventricular shunt surgery. *Child's Brain*, **7**, 182–9.

McLaurin, R. L. (1973) Infected cerebrospinal fluid shunts. *Surg. Neurol.*, **1**, 191–5.

Meers, P. D. (1983a) Ventilation in operating rooms. *Br. Med. J.*, **286**, 244–5.

Meers, P. D. (1983b) Ventilation in operating rooms. *Br. Med. J.*, **286**, 1215.

Michael, A. F., Drummond, K. N., Good, R. A. and Vernier, R. L. (1966) Acute post-streptococcal glomerulonephritis: Immune deposit disease. *J. Clin. Invest.*, **45**, 237–48.

von Moltz, G. and Doswald, T. (1976) Diffuse Glomerulonephritis bei Staphylokokken-infizierter ventrikuloatrialer Liquor Drainage. *Schweiz. Arch. Neurol. Neurochir. Psychiatr.*, **107**, 223–30.

Moncrieff, M. W., Glasgow, E. F., Arthur, L. J. H. and Hargreaves, H. M. (1973) Glomerulonephritis associated with *Staphylococcus albus* in a Spitz–Holter valve. *Arch. Dis. Child.*, **48**, 69–72.

Morrice, J. J. and Young, D. G. (1974) Bacterial colonisation of Holter valves: a ten year survey. *Dev. Med. Child. Neurol.*, (Suppl.) **32**, 85–90.

Moss, S. W., Gary, N. E. and Eissinger, R. P. (1977) Nephritis associated with a diphtheroid-infected cerebrospinal fluid shunt. *Am. J. Med.*, **63** (2), 318–19.

Myers, M. G. and Schoenbaum, S. C. (1975) Shunt fluid aspiration. *Am. J. Dis. Child.*, **129**, 220–2.

Newman, R. L. and Holt, R. J. (1967) Intrathecal gentamicin in treatment of ventriculitis in children. *Br. Med. J.*, **2**, 539–42.

Newman, R. L. and Holt, R. J. (1971) Gentamicin in paediatrics. I. Report on intrathecal gentamicin. *J. Infect. Dis.*, **124**, (Suppl. s), 254–6.

Nicholas, J. L., Kamal, I. M. and Eckstein, H. B. (1970) Immediate shunt replacement in the treatment of bacterial colonisation of Holter valves. *Dev. Med. Child. Neurol.*, **12**, (Suppl. 22) 110–13.

Nishino, T. and Nakazawa, S. (1976) Bacteriological study on effects of beta-lactam group antibiotics in high concentrations. *Antimicrob. Agents Chemother.*, **9**, 1033–42.

Nitti, V., Virgillio, R., Patricolo, M. R. and Juliano, A. (1977) Pharmacokinetic study of intravenous rifampicin. *Chemotherapy*, **23**, 1–6.

Noble, R. C. and Cooper, R. M. (1977) Gonococcal meningitis and ventriculitis in the presence of a ventriculoperitoneal shunt. *Sex. Transm. Dis.*, **4**, 9–11.

Noble, W. C. (1981) In *Microbiology of Human Skin*, 2nd edn, Lloyd Luke, London.

Noble, W. C. and Somerville, D. A. (1974) *Microbiology of Human Skin*. Saunders, Philadelphia.

Nolan, C. M., Flanigan, W. J., Rastogi, S. P. and Brewer, T. E. (1980) Vancomycin penetration into CSF during treatment of patients receiving haemodialysis. *South. Med. J.*, **73** (10), 1333–4.

Nosik, W. A. (1950) Ventriculomastoidostomy: Technique and observations. *J. Neurosurg.*, **7**, 236–9.

Nulsen, F. E. and Becker, D. P. (1965) Control of hydrocephalus by valve-regulated shunt. *J. Neurosurg.*, **26**, 363–74.

Nulsen, F. E. and Spitz, E. (1951) Treatment of hydrocephalus by direct shunt from ventricle to jugular vein. *Surg. Forum*, **2**, 399–403.

O'Brien, M., Parent, A. and Davis, B. (1979) Management of ventricular shunt infections. *Child's Brain*, **5**, 304–9.

Odio, C., Mohs, E., Sklar, F. H. *et al.* (1984) Adverse reactions to vancomycin used as prophylaxis for CSF shunt procedures. *Am. J. Dis. Child.*, **138**, 17–19.

Olsen, L., Grotte, G. and Nordbring, F. (1977) Successful treatment of *Pseudomonas aeruginosa* ventriculitis with intraventricular gentamicin in a child with hydrocephalus. *Scand. J. Infect. Dis.*, **9**, 243–5.

O'Regan, S. and Makker, S. P. (1979) Shunt nephritis: demonstration of diphtheroid antigen in glomeruli. *Am J. Med. Sci.*, **278** (2), 161–5.

Overton, M. C., Kirksey, T. D., Snodgrass, S. R. *et al.* (1967) Direct atrial and vena caval shunting procedures for hydrocephalus. *Surg. Gynecol. Obstet.*, **124**, 819–825.

Overton, M. C. and Snodgrass, S. R. (1965) Ventriculovenous shunts for infantile hydrocephalus. *J. Neurosurg.*, **23**, 517–21.

Parry, S. W., Schumaker, J. F. and Llewellyn, R. C. (1975) Abdominal pseudocysts and ascites formation after ventriculoperitoneal shunt procedures: Report of four cases. *J. Neurosurg.*, **27**, 21–6.

Patriarca, P. A. and Lauer, B. A. (1980) Ventriculoperitoneal shunt-associated infection due to *Haemophilus influenzae*. *Pediatr.*, **65** (5), 1007–9.

Payr, E. (1908) Drainage eines Seitenventrikels bei Hydrocephalus internus. *Dtsch. Med. Wochenschr.*, 532–4.

Perrin, J. C. and McLaurin, R. L. (1967) Infected ventriculo–atrial shunts. A method of treatment. *J. Neurosurg.*, **27**, 21–6.

Peters, G., Locci, R. and Pulverer, G. (1981) Microbial colonisation of prosthetic devices II. Scanning elctron microscopy of naturally infected intravenous catheters. *Zentralbl. Bakteriol.* (Orig. B), **173**, 293–9.

Pinals, R. S. and Tunnessen, W. W. (1977) Shunt arthritis. *J. Pediatr.*, **91** (4), 681.

Porter, F. N. (1975) Hydrocephalus treated by compressive head wrapping. *Arch. Dis. Child.*, **50** (10), 816–18.

Price, P. B. (1951) Fallacy of a current surgical fad: the three-minute pre-operative scrub with hexachlorophane soap. *Ann. Surg.*, **134** (1), 475–85.

Pudenz, R., Russel, F. E., Hurd, A. H. and Sheldon, C. H. (1957) Ventriculo-auriculostomy: a technique for shunting cerebrospinal fluid into the right auricle. Preliminary report. *J. Neurosurg.*, **14**, 171–9.

Pui, C. H., Lawrence, T. C. and Vanderzwagg, R. (1981) Shunt-associated bacterial infections in hydrocephalic children. *Ala. J. Med. Sci.*, **18**, 134–7.

Puri, P. and Harvey, T. W. (1981) Colonisation of ventriculo–atrial shunt with *Brucella abortus*. *Br. Med. J.*, **282**, 1754–5.

Raahave, D. (1974) Bacterial density in operation wounds. *Acta Chir. Scand.*, **140** (8), 585–93.

Raahave, D. (1976) Effect of plastic skin and wound drapes on the density of bacteria in operation wounds. *Br. J. Surg.*, **63**, 421–6.

Raimondi, A. J., Robinson, J. S. and Kuwamara, K. (1977) Complications of ventriculoperitoneal shunting and a critical comparison of three-piece and one-piece systems. *Child's Brain*, **3**, 321–42.

Rames, L., Wise, B., Goodman, J. R. and Piel, C. F. (1970) Renal disease with *Staphylococcus albus* bacteraemia. *JAMA*, **212**, 1671–7.

Raoult, D., Kohler, J. L., Gallais, H. and Casanova, P. (1981) Septicemie a *Staphylocoque epidermidis* multiresistant avec localisation meningee. *Nouv. Presse Med.*, **10** (47), 3855–6.

Raphael, S. S. and Donaghue, M. (1976) Infection due to *Bacillus cereus*. *Can. Med. Assoc. J.*, **115** (3), 207.

Rapport, M. M., Schwartz, A. E. and Graf, L. (1957) C-reactive protein in patients following operation. *Ann. Surg.*, **145** (3), 321–5.

Rekate, H. L., Ruch, T. and Nulsen, F. E. (1980) Diphtheroid infections of cerebrospinal fluid shunts. The changing pattern of shunt infection in Cleveland. *J. Neurosurg.*, **52** (4), 553–6.

Rennels, M. B. and Wald, E. R. (1980) Treatment of *Haemophilus influenzae* type b meningitis in children with cerebrospinal fluid shunts. *J. Pediatr.*, **97**, (3), 424–6.

Reynolds, M., Sherman, J. O. and Malone, D. G. (1983) Ventriculoperitoneal shunt infection masquerading as an acute surgical abdomen. *J. Pediatr. Surg.*, **18**, 951–4.

Riley, H. D. (1970) Vancomycin and novobiocin. *Med. Clin. North Am.*, **54**, 1277–89.

Ring, J. C., Cates, K. L., Belani, K. K. *et al.* (1979) Rifampicin for CSF shunt infections caused by coagulase-negative staphylococci. *J. Pediatr.*, **95** (2), 317–9.

Ring, P. A. (1974) Total replacement of hip joint. A review of a thousand operations. *J. Bone Joint. Surg.*, **56B** (1), 44–58.

Robertson, J. S., Maraqa, M. I. and Jennett, B. (1973) Ventriculoperitoneal shunting for hydrocephalus. *Br. Med. J.*, **2**, 289–92.

Rodgers, B. M., Vries, J. K. and Talbert, J. L. (1978) Laparoscopy in the diagnosis and treatment of malfunctioning ventriculoperitoneal shunts in children. *J. Pediatr. Surg.*, **13** (3), 247–53.

Ryan, J. L., Pachner, A., Andriole, V. T. and Root, R. K. (1980) Enterococcal meningitis: combined vancomycin and rifampicin therapy. *Am. J. Med.*, **68** (3), 449–51.

Sabath, L. D., Garner, C. and Wilcox, C. (1976) Susceptibility of *Staphylococcus aureus* and *Staphylococcus epidermidis* to 65 antibiotics. *Antimicrob. Agents Chemother.*, **9**, 962–9.

Saggers, B. A. and Stewart, G. T. (1964) Polyvinylpyrrolidone iodine: an assessment of antibacterial activity. *J. Hyg. (Camb.)*, **62**, 509–18.

Salmon, J. H. (1972) Adult hydrocephalus: evaluation of shunt therapy in 80 patients. *J. Neurosurg.*, **37**, 423–8.

Schaad, U. B., McCracken, G. H. and Nelson, J. D. (1980) Clinical pharmacology and efficacy of vancomycin in pediatric patients. *J. Pediatr.*, **96**, 119–26.

Schimke, R. T., Black, P. H., Mark, V. H. and Schwartz, M. N. (1961) Indolent *Staphylococcus albus* or *aureus* bacteraemia after ventriculo-atriostomy. *N. Engl. J. Med.*, **264**, 264–70.

Schleifer, K. H. and Kloos, W. E. (1975) A simple test system for separation of staphylococci from micrococci. *J. Clin. Microbiol.*, **1** (3), 337–8.

Schlesinger, J. J. and Ross, A. L. (1977) *Propionibacterium acnes* meningitis in a previously normal adult. *Arch. Intern. Med.*, **37** (7), 921–3.

Schoenbaum, S. C., Gardner, P. and Shillito, J. (1975) Infections of cerebrospinal fluid shunts: epidemiology, clinical manifestations and therapy. *J. Infect. Dis.*, **131** (5), 543–52.

Sells, C. J., Shurtleff, D. B. and Loesser, J. D. (1977) Gram-negative cerebrospinal fluid shunt-associated infections. *Pediatr.*, **59** (4), 614–18.

Shibolet, S., Dan, M., Jedwab, M. *et al.* (1979) Recurrent miliary tuberculosis secondary to infected ventriculo–atrial shunt. *Chest*, **76** (3), 328–30.

Shooter, R. A., Smith, M. A., Griffiths, J. D. *et al.* (1958) Spread of staphylococcus in a surgical ward. *Br. Med. J.*, **5071**, 607–613.

Shurtleff, D. B., Foltz, E. L. and Christie, D. (1971) Ventriculoauriculostomy-associated infection: A 12-year study. *J. Neurosurg.*, **35**, 686–94.

Shurtleff, D. B., Foltz, E. L., Weeks, R. D. and Loesser, J. (1974) Therapy of *Staphylococcus epidermidis*: infections associated with cerebrospinal fluid shunts. *Pediatr.*, **53**, 52–62.

Skinner, P. R., Taylor, A. J. and Coakham, H. (1978) Propionibacteria as a cause of shunt and post neurosurgical infections. *J. Clin. Pathol.*, **31** (11), 1085–9.

Smith, I. M., Beals, P. D., Kingsbury, K. R. and Hasenclever, H. F. (1958) Observations on *Staphylococcus albus* septicaemia in mice and men. *AMA Arch. Intern. Med.*, **102**, 375–88.

Spector, R. and Lorenzo, A. V. (1974) Inhibition of penicillin transport from the cerebrospinal fluid after intracisternal inoculation of bacteria. *J. Clin. Invest.*, **54**, 316–25.

Stamey, T. A. and Condy, M. (1975) The diffusion and concentration of trimethoprim in human vaginal fluid. *J. Infect. Dis.*, **131**, 261–6.

Stauffer, U. G. (1970) Shunt nephritis, a complication of ventriculo–atrial shunts. *Dev. Med. Child. Neurol.*, **12**, (Suppl. 22), 161–4.

Stern, S., Bayston, R. and Hayward, R. J. (1988) *Haemophilus influenzae* meningitis in the presence of cerebrospinal fluid shunts. *Child's Nerv. Syst.*, **3** (in press).

Stickler, G. B., Skin, M. H., Burke, E. C. *et al.* (1968) Diffuse glomerulonephritis associated with infected ventriculoatrial shunt. *N. Engl. J. Med.*, **20**, 1077–82.

Story, P. (1952) Testing of skin disinfectants. *Br. Med. J.*, **ii**, 1128–30.

Strife, C. F., McDonald, B. M., Ruley, E. J. *et al.* (1976) Shunt nephritis: the nature of serum cryoglobulins and their relation to the complement profile. *J. Pediatr.*, **88** (3), 403–13.

Strominger, J. L. and Tipper, D. J. (1965) Bacterial cell wall synthesis and structure in relation to the mechanism of action of penicillins and other antibacterial agents. *Am. J. Med.*, **39**, 708–21.

Sugarman, B. (1982) *In vitro* adherence of bacteria to prosthetic vascular grafts. *Infection*, **10** (1), 9/13–12/16.

Sutherland, G. E., Palitang, E. G., Marr, J. J. and Lwedke, S. L. (1981) Sterilisation of Ommaya reservoir by installation of vancomycin. *Am. J. Med.*, **71**, 1068–70.

Suwanwela, C. (1968) Complications of tuberculous meningitis. *Proc. Aust. Assoc. Neurol.*, **5**, 493–5.

Swayne, R., Rampling, A. and Newsom, S. W. B. (1987) Intraventricular vancomycin for treatment of shunt-associated ventriculitis. *J. Antimicrob. Chemother.*, **19**, 249 53.

Tabara, Z., Azmy, A. and Forrest, D. M. (1980) Direct atriotomy. *Z. Kinderchir.*, **31** (4), 359–62.

Tabara, Z. and Forrest, D. M. (1982) Colonisation of CSF shunts: preventative measures. *Z. Kinderchir.*, **37** (4), 156–8.

Tillet, W. S. and Francis, T. (1930) Serological reactions in pneumonia with a non-protein somatic fraction of pneumococcus. *J. Exp. Med.*, **52**, 561–71.

Toala, P., McDonald, A. and Wilcox, C. (1969) Susceptibility of Group D streptococcus (enterococcus) to 21 antibiotics *in vitro*, with special reference to species differences. *Am. J. Med. Sci.*, **258**, 416–30.

Traub, W. H. (1981) Variable tolerance of a clinical isolate of *Staphylococcus epidermidis* from an infected hydrocephalus shunt for several beta-lactam antibiotics, vancomycin and fosfomycin. *Chemotherapy*, **27**, 432–43.

Tschirgi, R. D., Frost, R. W. and Taylor, J. L. (1954) Inhibition of cerebrospinal fluid formation by a carbonic anhydride inhibitor, 2-acetyl-amino-1, 3, 4, -thiadiazole-5-sulphonamide (Diamox). *Proc. Soc. Exp. Biol. Med.*, **87**, 373–6.

Tsingoglou, S. and Forrest, D. M. (1968) Therapeutic and prophylactic lengthening of distal catheter of the Holter ventriculo–atrial shunt. *Dev. Med. Child. Neurol.*, **10**, (suppl. 16), 35–43.

Tsingoglou, S. and Forrest, D. M. (1971a) A technique for the insertion of Holter ventriculo–atrial shunt for infantile hydrocephalus. *Br. J. Surg.*, **58** (5), 367–72.

Tsingoglou, S. and Forrest, D. M. (1971b) Complications from Holter ventriculo–atrial shunts. *Br. J. Surg.*, **58** (5), 372–7.

Upadhyaya, P., Bhargava. S., Sundaram, K. R. *et al.* (1983) Hydrocephalus caused by tuberculous meningitis: clinical picture, CT findings and results of shunt surgery. *Z. Kinderchir.*, **38**, (Suppl. II), 76–80.

Valenton, M. J. and Okumoto, M. (1973) Toxin-producing strains of *Staphylococcus epidermidis (albus)*. Isolates from patients with Staphylococcic blepharoconjunctivitis. *Arch. Ophthalmol.*, **89**, 186–9.

Velghe, L., Dereymaeker, A. and van der Voorde, H. (1964) Swabbing of operative field in neurosurgery: Analysis of 1000 controls. *Acta Neurosurg. (Wien)*, **II**, 686–93.

Venes, J. L. (1976) Control of shunt infection: Report of 150 consecutive cases. *J. Neurosurg.*, **45**, 311–14.

Verhoef, F. J., Winkler, K. C. and van Boven, C. P. A. (1971) Lysogeny in coagulase-negative staphylococci. *J. Med. Microbiol.*, **4**, 405–12.

Villarejo, F. J. (1979) Post operative ventriculitis in hydrocephalus. *Acta Neurochir. (Wien)*, **48** (1–2), 41–5.

Visconti, E. B. and Peters, G. (1979) Vancomycin treatment of cerebrospinal fluid shunt infections. Report of two cases. *J. Neurosurg.*, **51** (2), 245–6.

Wake, P. N., Humphrey, C. and Walker, R. (1980) Longterm intravenous rifampicin after massive small bowel resection. *Tubercle*, **61**, 109–11.

Wald, S. L. and McLaurin, R. L. (1978) Shunt-associated glomerulonephritis. *Neurosurg.*, **3** (2), 146–50.

Wasson, K. R. and Harris, J. O. (1976) The treatment of tuberculosis in the presence of malabsorption syndromes. *Amer. Rev. Respir. Dis.*, **113**, 51.

Watanakunakorn, C. (1978) Antibiotic-tolerant *Staphylococcus aureus*. *J. Antimicrob. Chemother.*, **4**, 561–8.

Watanakunakorn, C. (1981) The antibacterial action of vancomycin. *Rev. Inf. Dis.*, **3** (Suppl.), 210–5.

Watanakunakorn, C. and Guerriero, J. C. (1981) Interaction between vancomycin and rifampicin against *Staphylococcus aureus*. *Antimicrob. Agents Chemother.*, **19** (6), 1089–91.

Weinstein, M. P., La Force, F. M., Mangi, R. J. and Quintiliani, R. (1977) Non-pneumococcal gram-positive coccal meningitis related to neurosurgery. *J. Neurosurg.*, **47** (2), 236–40.

Welch, K. (1977) The prevention of shunt infection. *Z. Kinderchir.*, **22**, 465–75.

Wichman, S., Von König, C. H. W., Becker-Boost, E. and Finger, H. (1984) Isolation of corynebacterium Group JK from clinical specimens with a semi-selective medium. *J. Clin. Microbiol.*, **19** (2), 204–6.

Wilson, C. B. and Pertan, V. (1966) Perforation of the bowel complicating peritoneal shunt for hydrocephalus. Report of two cases. *Am. Surg.*, **32**, 601–3.

Wise, B. L., Mathis, J. L. and Wright, J. H. (1966) Experimental use of isosorbide; an oral osmotic agent to lower cerebrospinal fluid pressure and reduce brain bulk. *J. Neurosurg.*, **25**, 183–8.

Young, E. J., Ratner, R. E. and Clarridge, J. E. (1981) Staphylococcal ventriculitis treated with vancomycin. *South. Med. J.*, **74** (8), 1014–15.

Yu, H. C. and Patterson, R. H. (1973) Prophylactic antimicrobial agents after ventriculostomy for hydrocephalus. *J. Pediatr. Surg.*, **8** (6), 881–5.

INDEX

Acetazolamide 1
Acute abdomen, in
    ventriculoperitoneal shunt
    infections 37, 62
Adhesion of organisms to shunt
    material 15
Adhesions, peritoneal 52, 55, 56
Airborne bacteria, and shunt
    infections 29–30, 126
Air ventriculogram 50
Aminoglycosides 114–17
Anaemia, in ventriculo–atrial shunt
    infections 59, 60, 65
Antibacterial catheters 139–40
Antibiotic cover for dental surgery
    139
Antibiotic prophylaxis 131–8
    recommended 140
Antibody to coagulase-negative
    staphylococci 78–82
    age related titres 81
    common antigen 79
    delay in appearance 81
    method 79–80
    persistence of raised titres 82
    rationale 78–9
    test, interpretation of results
        80–2, 92–4
Antimicrobial wound packs 130–1
Arthralgia, in shunt infections 63,
    66
Ascending infection
    due to ruptured appendix 26
    due to visceral perforation 26, 54
    in Spina Bifida 42

Bacillus spp.
    shunt infection 40–1
    toxic demyelination 41
Bacteraemia 11, 23–6
Bacteriological typing and
    identification methods 31–5

Bacteroides, in shunt infection 42,
    48–9
Biocompatibility 2
Blood cultures
    capillary 68
    contamination 68–9
    in ventriculo–atrial shunt
        infections 68
    in ventriculoperitoneal shunt
        infections 52
    postoperative 28
Brucella, in shunt infections 44

Candida, in shunt infections 44–5,
    51
Cardiac shunts, direct 2
Ceftriaxone 110–11
Cefuroxime 109
Cell wall active antimicrobials
    109–10
Cephalothin 98
Chloramphenicol 104, 105, 111–12,
    120, 121
Chlorhexidine 43, 131
    contamination with
        Pseudomonas 43
Choice of antimicrobials, rationale
    108
Classification of shunt infections
    13, 77, 131
Clindamycin, in prophylaxis 134
Clinical features of shunt infections
    58–60
Cloxacillin 109, 123
Coagulase-negative staphylococci
    bacteriophage typing 31
    biotyping 31
    nomenclature 13
    sensityping 32–3
    slime production 15–23
Coliforms, in shunt infections 42,
    49, 54

Compressive head bandaging 1
Comparison of ventriculo–atrial
    and ventriculoperitoneal
    shunts 12–13, 59–62
Coryneforms
  in shunt infections 19, 31, 33–7,
    117
  JK group 34, 117
  shunt nephritis due to 35
Co-trimoxazole 112–13
  rash due to 113
C-reactive protein 82–7
  effects of antibiotics 81, 93
  in cerebrospinal fluid 86
  in external shunt infections 58, 85
    shunt nephritis 63, 65, 85, 86
    ventriculo–atrial shunt
      infections 81–6
    ventriculoperitoneal shunt
      infections 52, 61, 84, 86
  other causes of positive results
    82–5
  related to surgery 83–4
  tests for 86–7
Cystic blockage of
    ventriculoperitoneal shunts
    51–7, 86, 93

Depilatory cream 129
Diagnosis
  of infective blockage 56
  of shunt infection 58–89
Disseminated intravascular
    coagulation 58–9
Dissemination of infection by
    shunting 45–6, 105
Distal catheter colonization 71
Drapes, surgical 129–30, 131

'Early' and 'late' shunt infections
    23–7, 92
Electrolyte loss 2
Erosion of skin over shunt 26, 44, 58
Erythema over shunt 58
Examination of removed shunts
    72–8, 99
External shunt colonization 13, 58,
    77, 126, 131
External ventricular drainage 54,
    97, 103
Extracellular slime 15–23, 79

Flucloxacillin 123
Fusidic acid 123

Gallium scan, in
    ventriculoperitoneal shunt
    infection 56
Gentamicin, intraventricular 102,
    112, 116, 120, 124
  cerebrospinal fluid levels 102, 116
  complications 102, 116–17, 136–7
  dose 117
Gentamicin wound packs 130

Hawthorn effect 133
Haematogenous seeding, theory of
    23–6
Haematuria, *see* Shunt nephritis
Haemophilus meningitis in shunted
    patients 47, 103–5
Hexachlorophane 128, 131
Hydrocephalus
  causes 1
  definition 1
  drug treatment 1
  neurological damage due to 1

Imersion of shunts before insertion
    130–1, 136, 137
Immediate shunt replacement for
    infection 105–7
Immune complex disease 66–8
Incarceration of organisms in
    blocked shunts 60
Incidence of shunt colonization 12,
    13
Internal shunt colonization 13, 126
Intraventricular antimicrobials
    97–102, 110, 137
Iodine 127
Iodophores 70, 127, 131
Isosorbide 1

JK coryneforms, *see* Coryneforms

Laparoscopy in
    ventriculoperitoneal shunt
    blockage 55
'Late' infections
  aetiology 26
  and shunt nephritis 65
Lengthening of ventriculo–atrial
    shunts 10

Listeria monocytogenes in shunt
infections 39–40, 117
Lumbar–peritoneal shunts 2

Methicillin 109
intraventricular 97, 98
prophylactic 132
Methotrexate, intraventricular,
compatibility with
vancomycin 120, 122
Metrizamide, and cerebrospinal
fluid pleocytosis 72
Microcolonies 15
Mixed infections 48–9, 54
Mode and time of entry of
colonizing organisms 23–7,
28–31, 57
Moraxella, in shunt infections 43
Mycobacterium spp. in shunt
infections, 45–6
risk of dissemination due to
shunting 46

Nafcillin 111, 120
Neisseria gonorrhoeae in shunt
infections 46, 104–5, 124
Neisseria meningitidis in shunt
infections 46, 104–5, 124
Netilmicin, intraventricular dose
124
Nocardia in shunt infections 40
Noxythiolin 130
Numerical antibiogram 32–3
Numerical biochemical profile 32

'Occult' shunt infections 78
Oral therapy 110–11

Patient's skin, as source of infecting
organisms 27–8
preparation for surgery 126–8
Penetration of antimicrobials into
cerebrospinal fluid 136
Penicillin 124
Peptococcus spp. in shunt infections
41
Perilymph, and ototoxicity 116
Period of risk of shunt infections
131
Peritoneal abscess 61
Peritonitis 61, 110

Phage typing, *see* Bacteriological
typing and identification
methods
Phagocytes and silicone rubber
22–3
Pneumococcal meningitis in
shunted patients 47, 105, 124
Pneumonopathy 67
Povidone iodine 127, 131, 137
Preoperative preparation of
patient's skin 126–8, 131, 137
recommended 140
shaving 128–9
Prevention of shunt infections
126–40
Probenecid 108
Programmable (adjustable) shunts
3, 4
Prophylaxis for shunt operations
131–8
Propionibacterium species in shunt
infections 37–9
and shunt nephritis 38
Pseudomonas species in shunt
infections 42–3, 59
Pulmonary embolus 60

Quinolones, 123

Radiocontrast studies for shunt
patency 51–6
Rash 63, 66–7
Reflux and ascending infection 25–6
Renal biopsy for diagnosis of shunt
nephritis 67
Reservoir
Ommaya 120
Rickham 3, 124
Resident skin flora 127
Retrograde extension of shunt
infections 50
'Rhodochrous Complex', *see*
Nocardia
Rifampicin 110, 113–14, 120–1
dose 125
Rifampin, *see* Rifampicin
Routes of shunting 1, 2

Serological diagnosis of shunt
infection 78–7

Serological surveillance for shunt
  infection 65, 90–6
Serratia spp. in shunt infections 43
Shunt aspiration 50, 70–1, 72
Shunt insertion techniques 4–10
  lengthening 10
  removal for infection 102–7
    complications of 103
  revision 10–11
Shunt nephritis 11, 35, 38, 39–40,
    41, 60, 86, 111, 118
  and delayed diagnosis 86, 89, 94,
    95
  and ventriculoperitoneal shunts
    62, 65–6
  pathogenesis 62–3
  prevention 65, 94, 95
  serological diagnosis 63–5, 88
  serum complement levels in 65,
    67, 88
Shunt obstruction, due to candida
    45
Skin flora 27
Slime, *see* Extracellular slime
Sources of infecting organisms
    27–31
Splenomegaly 59, 60, 64
Staphylococcus aureus shunt
    infections 18, 19, 21, 60, 62
  antialpha toxin 58
  clinical features 62
  disseminated intravascular
    coagulation in 58–9
Staphylococcus epidermidis, see
    Coagulase-negative
    staphylococci
Streptococcus pneumoniae
    meningitis in shunted
    patients 47, 105, 124
Streptococcus spp. in shunt

infections 48
Sulphonamides 110
Surgical expertise and experience
    30–1, 131, 133, 136, 140

Teicoplanin 117, 122
Thrombosis
  sinus 2
  venous 60
Treatment of shunt infections
    96–124
  non surgical versus surgical
    97–102
  randomized trial 100–1
  recommendations 123–4
Trimethoprim 110, 112–13, 123, 125

Vancomycin 117–25
  intravenous 118–19
  intraventricular 119–22, 124, 138
  used with rifampicin 120
Ventriculitis 50, 106, 107, 110
  persisting 61, 106
  spontaneous resolution 110
  treatment 110, 119
Ventriculo–atrial shunt infections,
    clinical features 60
Ventriculocardiac shunts, direct 2
Ventriculoperitoneal shunt
    infections
  clinical features 52, 61
  cystic blockage 51–7
Ventriculoperitoneal shunts 2, 85
Ventriculo–ureteral shunts 99
Visceral perforation by shunt tubing
    54, 100
  following non–surgical treatment
    of infection 49, 116

Wound infections 131